100

NATURAL

BEAUTY

TIPS

THAT WILL MAKE YOU
BEAUTIFUL FOREVER

Contents

> *"The beauty of a woman is not in the clothes she wears, the figure that she carries, or the way she combs her hair. The beauty of a woman is seen in her eyes, because that is the doorway to her heart, the place where love resides. True beauty in a woman is reflected in her soul. It's the caring that she lovingly gives, the passion that she shows & the beauty of a woman only grows with passing years."*
>
> *— Audrey Hepburn*

Beauty today is not about the latest trends, a certain stereotype or being something that you are not. Beauty starts from within, your body is a gift and it is your responsibility to honor and respect it. Beauty is about making the most of your natural assets so that you feel more confident and positive about whom you are.

Eating well, exercising and using the right skincare are essential ingredients to making the most of your own true beauty. However there are other insider tips that can give you a little beauty boost and empower you to own your own unique beauty.

This book will empower you to find your own authentic beauty, no matter your age or circumstance. Every page reveals a sacred beauty tip, as you turn each page you will slowly unveil the mystique of beauty, you will be taken on a journey to discovering your own "true beauty".

This book is an indispensable beauty guide, over flowing with top-to-toe beauty tips, tricks and treatments. And as a bonus, at the end of this book there is a 21 day plan which will change the way you look and feel.

Remember that true beauty is ageless, it is not about the wrinkles or dress size. True beauty is about taking care of yourself and living with love in your heart. Let this book guide you to be inspired so that you live life to the fullest by making the most of your body, your looks and most of all yourself.

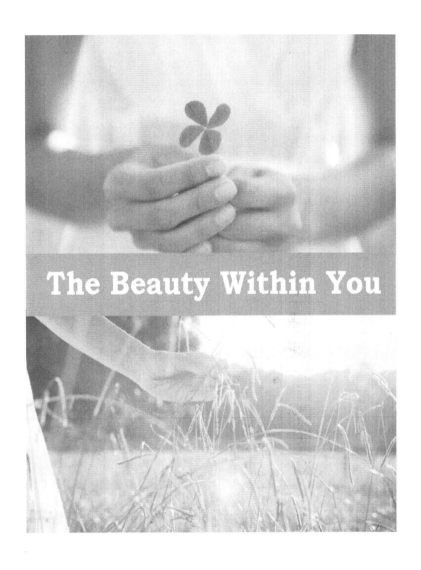

The Beauty Within You

Rediscovering your true authentic self

"I am Me. In all the world, there is no one else exactly like me. Everything that comes out of me is authentically mine, because I alone chose it -- I own everything about me: my body, my feelings, my mouth, my voice, all my actions, whether they be to others or myself. I own my fantasies, my

dreams, my hopes, my fears. I own my triumphs and successes, all my failures and mistakes. Because I own all of me, I can become intimately acquainted with me. By so doing, I can love me and be friendly with all my parts. I know there are aspects about myself that puzzle me, and other aspects that I do not know -- but as long as I am friendly and loving to myself, I can courageously and hopefully look for solutions to the puzzles and ways to find out more about me. However, I look and sound, whatever I say and do, and whatever I think and feel at a given moment in time is authentically me. If later some parts of how I looked, sounded, thought, and felt turn out to be unfitting, I can discard that which is unfitting, keep the rest, and invent something new for that which I discarded. I can see, hear, feel, think, say, and do. I have the tools to survive, to be close to others, to be productive, and to make sense and order out of the world of people and things outside of me. I own me, and therefore, I can engineer me. I am me, and I am Okay." ~ Virginia Satir

In a world that is incredibly loud it is easy to lose yourself in the noise and forget who you truly are. It is all too common for many people to disconnect from their true essence and live a life that is not their truth. The art to finding true beauty is truly knowing and accepting oneself. To get started we are going to delve a little deeper into who you really are.

Take a moment to get to know yourself, forget about the world and what other people expect from you. Ask yourself these questions. What would you like to improve? What are your goals? Would you like glossier hair? A more toned body? More energy? Better health? A happier outlook?

By answering these questions truthfully, you should have a rough idea on what you want in your life and what you need to improve. It is extremely important to drop all judgment that you hold of yourself right now. You need to get proactive and create goals and steps to achieve what you want. You need to stay positive to allow yourself to find solutions to situations instead of allowing yourself to be held back by that same old negative attitude that you established years ago.

It is time to become aware of all your self-limiting beliefs and excuses that have held you back long enough. It is time to stop labeling yourself as 'weak' or 'just not good enough'. You need to replace these thoughts with positive affirmations. From today forward you need to believe that it is within your power to achieve whatever it is you desire. You can change anything if you want to.

It's now time to turn those old self-limiting beliefs into positive thought patterns. Get out your notebook and write down all your strengths. Then make a list of all your weaknesses. Turn your weaknesses into a positive by writing an affirmation for each weakness. When you write an affirmation you need to have it written as if it has already happened. For example if you want to lose weight, don't write "I want to lose weight". An effective affirmation would be "I am fit and healthy".

Changing your though patterns is the first key to changing yourself. Positive thinking will give you the ammunition and energy to achieve whatever it is that you crave.

It is never too late to change thought patterns and start investing in yourself. Living well by looking after yourself is not self-indulgent – it is simply living the best you can for as long as you can.

The art of true beauty = To discover yourself is to learn about yourself. To learn about yourself is to become aware of yourself. To become aware of yourself is to accept yourself. To accept yourself is to care for yourself. To care for yourself is to better yourself. To better yourself is to love yourself. To love yourself is to love the world. To love the world is to make the world a better place. To make the world a better place is the art of true beauty.

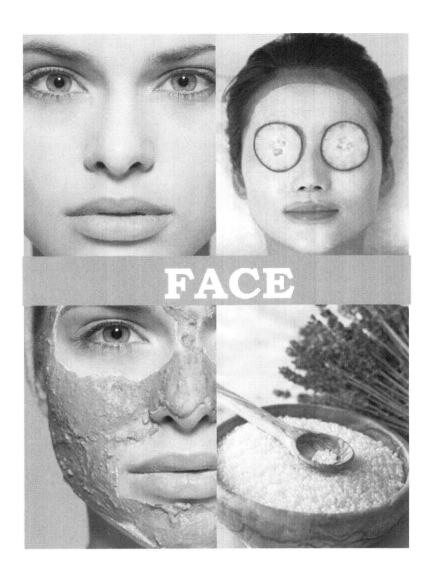

1. Face Mapping.

What is your skin trying to tell you? Face mapping is the art of unlocking the mysteries of your skin to help you treat pimples, adult acne, blemishes and other skin irritations.

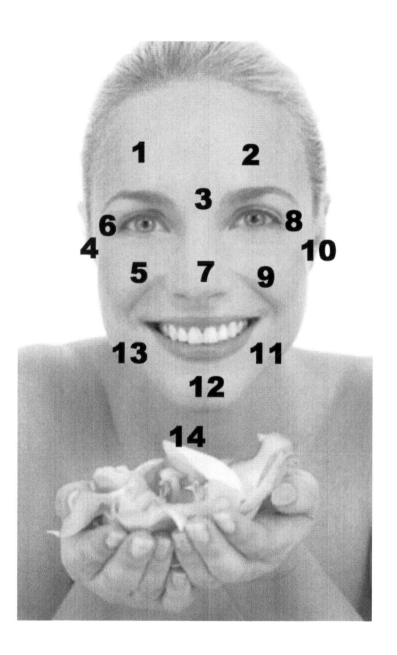

Nine times out of ten there is a solution behind your skin disorders. For example sudden breakouts around the mouth are typically caused by a hormonal imbalance – this is referred to as hormonal acne. Hormonal acne typically only occurs on the lower half of the face especially around the chin, mouth and jaw line Women are most susceptible to hormonal acne as things like the monthly cycle, contraception and pregnancy can all disrupt the delicate balance of hormones.

Hormonal break outs can be quite obvious because they frequently appear as papules on the skins surface. Papules are solid raised pimples. The breakout occurs because the hormones are producing excess oil.

So, what are your breakouts, spots and dark circles trying to tell you? Here's a quick guide:

The Zones	The Reasons Behind
Zone 1 & 3:	Bladder & Digestive System — Improve your diet by eating more wholefoods and hydrate with at least two liters of water a day.
Zone 2:	Liver — Slow down party girl. Try cutting back on alcohol, heavy foods or dairy. This area can also indicate a food allergy.
Zone 4 & 10:	Kidneys — Keep yourself hydrated with water and toss the caffeine and soda.
Zone 5 & 9:	Respiratory system — This area tends to break out in acne with people who smoke or have allergies.
Zone 6 & 8	Kidneys — Dark circles are usually a result of dehydration. Drink more water and less caffeine!
Zone 7:	Heart — Take some time to chill out and find your bliss. Make sure you keep a check on your blood pressure.

Zone 12:	Stomach — It is time to clean up and renew - consider a detox to remove the toxins. You may also want to consider adding more fiber to your diet to help with digestion.
Zone 11 & 13:	Hormones — Stress and hormonal changes can sometimes be alleviated with more water, more sleep and a few extra servings of dark, leafy greens. If breakouts in this area are persistent, make an appointment with your doctor to look into a possible hormonal imbalance. Additionally, breakouts in this area can also indicate when you are ovulating.
Zone 14:	Illness — Can be a sign of your body fighting bacteria to avoid illness. Take some time out and drink plenty of fluids.

Face mapping is a traditional Chinese medicine, and is used by many holistic skincare experts. Your life events are often written and mapped on your face; therefore it is a great resource to use in analyzing your health and wellbeing and to pick up any imbalances within your body. Make an effort to study your face zones every couple of days, and within a few weeks you should see an improvement in your skin and overall health.

2. Boost Your Lashes.

Instead of paying a fortune for intensive lash treatments you can create your own treatment that is bursting with nourishment. To help thicken and lengthen your lashes simply apply coconut oil or almond oil to your lashes. A great way to do this is keep an old mascara wand, wash it and let it dry. Use the dry mascara wand to apply the nourishing oils to your lashes. It is a great idea to apply before bed so that all the goodness gets absorbed while you sleep.

"Beauty is not in the face; beauty is a light in the heart." - Kahlil Gibran

3. Eyebrow Perfection.

Eyebrows are the most defining feature of your face – they frame your eyes. You need to tread lightly when altering your eyebrows as the mistake of one over-plucked hair can lead to major eyebrow mishaps.

For eyebrow perfection follow these insider secrets:

- Cleanse the eyebrow area first.
- Hold a pencil flat along the side of your nose, aligning the corner of the nose and the tear duct. This is where your eyebrows should start. Then move the pencil to align the corner of the nose with the outer corner of the eye- this is where your eyebrow should end.

- Start at the middle of the brow and work outwards, removing a continuous line of hairs, one at a time.
- Always pluck hairs one line at a time underneath the brow, then stand back and glance at your overall look before plucking another line.

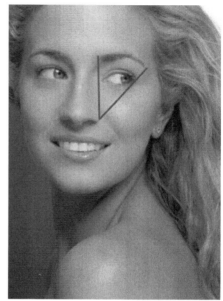

- Follow the natural shape of your eyebrows. Your eye shape will naturally determine what shape eyebrows suit your face best - whether you should go really thin, or retain a slightly fuller feel.
- Get a more defined look by filling in patchy sections with an eyebrow pencil. Use broken movements to keep the effect looking natural, stick to an eyebrow pencil about one shade lighter than your eyebrows.

"A Smile is the best makeup for any girl" – Unknown

4. Steam Clean Your Face

You need to steam clean your face at least once a week to remove blackheads, dirt, blemishes and unwanted toxins. The moisture from the steam helps to plump up dehydrated skin cells, giving you a youthful glow. Experts claim that the heat can stimulate certain facial muscles, leading to fewer lines and wrinkles.

How to give yourself a facial steam

Fill a large bowl with boiling water. Let the bowl stand for 5 minutes, as a gentle heat is all that is needed. For a little boost add a handful of herbs or a few drops of essential oil.

- Place a medium-sized towel over your head and neck and then lean forward over the bowl.
- Close your eyes and relax. Steam for about 10 - 15 minutes.
- Pat your skin dry with a clean towel and apply a nourishing moisturizer.

Herbs for your skin type:

Normal to dry skin – Lavender and chamomile essential oils.

Normal to oily skin – A few sprigs of fresh mint and a slice of lemon

Dry Skin – Evening primrose oil or jojoba carrier oil.

5. Soothe Tired And Puffy Eyes

Do you wake up with tired and puffy eyes? Here are a few things that can help soothe your eyes.

- Always remove your eye make-up before bed.
- Drink at least two liters of water a day to help flush out toxins and prevent fluid retention.

- Take care when applying eye cream. Make sure you gently dab the cream around the eye and not rub. Be careful to not get too close to your eye.
- If you do wake up with puffy eyes and you want to reduce the puffy effect then gently apply some cooling eye gel. Massage around the eye area working outwards. Place cucumber slices or cold chamomile teabags on eyes for 20 minutes.
- Puffy eyes are often caused from fluid retention and can be made worse by lying flat at night. Try changing your sleeping position. Add an extra pillow to help prevent fluids 'pooling'.

Blissful moments. *If you are feeling a little stressed, soak a face flannel in a bowl of warm water with 3 drops of lavender oil. Wring out the cloth, lie yourself down and place the flannel on your forehead. Breathe deeply and relax.*

6. Pimple Remedy

Oh no it is the night before a night out and you look in the mirror to only be greeted with a huge ugly pimple. Temptation is calling, you want to squeeze it. Whatever you do, do not be seduced by the temptation, it will only make the pimple worse. Here are some things you can do to help it.

- Only squeeze if the pimple is white. Use a warm clean face clothe and gently squeeze it.
- Wipe over the pimple with tea tree oil to kill any germs and infection.

- If you have redness a small wipe of lavender oil will help soothe this.
- Apply some raw honey on the pimple and leave overnight. You can cover with a small plaster so that the honey does not go everywhere.
- If you don't do the honey then apply a small clay mask over the pimple to help draw out the impurities.
- The next morning apply a blemish gel to help soothe and restore the infected area.

7. Clean Your Face

Cleaning your face and removing your make up before bed is a must. I know it can be hard to stick to this when you have had a super stressful day and it is late. Believe me when I say it is amazing how much residue and crap gets clogged in your skin, and if it is not removed it will make your skin look dull and lifeless. Here are some reasons why cleaning your face every night will give you a beauty boost:

- Cleansing removes the residue of the day, which often gets stuck in your pores causing more blackheads.
- Daily face washing helps the natural exfoliation process by removing excess skin and buffing the skin to a radiant shine. This brightens skin and diminishes fine lines, wrinkles and blemishes.

Beauty Tip- *Olive oil or coconut oil is a wonderful cleanser that will also feed your skin with vitamins and goodness.*

When cleaning your face never be over-zealous. A good product will leave your skin clean without excess rubbing. If your skin is acne prone, go gentler on cleansing. Clean your face morning and night – your skin will thank you for it.

8. Treat Rosacea

Rosacea is a fairly common skin disorder in which the nose, cheeks, forehead, or chin are affected. Rosacea can look like acne but isn't. Unlike acne, rosacea doesn't produce the typical blackheads or whiteheads and is more likely to be a problem after adolescents. Rosacea cannot be cured, but it can be soothed. Here are some ways that can help:

- Eating a diet rich in essential fatty acids will help reduce inflammation of the skin. Taking fish oil, flaxseed oil or hemp seed oil are all excellent sources of fatty acids.
- Loading up on your greens will help soothe the redness. By eating spirulina and your green vegetables, you are receiving a high supply of phytonutrients.
- Calm the inflammation with a cup of green tea which is full of healing properties.
- Avoid or reduce alcohol, coffee and spicy foods as they aggravate the skin.
- Reduce your exposure to the sun, wind and stress.
- Treat Rosacea naturally by applying pure Aloe Vera. The healing properties of this plant help reduce facial redness, whilst soothing and calming the skin. Aloe Vera also helps regenerate and heal skin tissue.
- Cleanse your face with 100% jojoba oil – it is amazing for rosacea. Jojoba oil contains essential omega 6 and 9 fatty acids and vitamins A, D and E in the perfect balance to support skin health. It has been used

through the ages to deep cleanse, moisture and condition all skin types.

Dry Skin? *Try an avocado face mask - simply apply avocado topically on your face, leave for 10 minutes and then rinse off with warm water.*

9. Be Sunscreen Savvy

UV radiation is the main cause of premature aging and uneven pigmentation. The best way to protect your skin is to use a face moisturizer or foundation that contains at least SPF 15. Always—no matter what season or climate you live in—wear sunscreen on your face, hands, and on any part of your skin that is exposed. Here are some facts about sunscreen that you need to know

- The SPF in your day creams and foundations provide what is called 'urban' protection. It is designed for minimal sun exposure. If you are spending more than 20 minutes outside it is recommended that you apply a stronger sunscreen.
- For maximum protection you need to reapply every two hours. Even sunscreens that state 'all day protection' need to be applied every two hours.
- Throw out your sunscreen every year and invest in a new tube. Whilst the expiry date is usually two years, it is wise to replace your sunscreen every year to ensure maximum protection.

A beauty tip. *Don't ban sunshine completely as a small dose of daily sunshine is good for your wellbeing. Sunshine infuses your body with Vitamin D which is known to reduce the risk of many cancers.*

10. Stop Premature Aging

The number one accessory for anyone to have is great skin. When your skin looks great you radiate health and vitality. At around the age of 25 your skin renewal starts to slow down, less oil is produced so your skin often feels drier and tighter. Cell renewal takes longer so your skin can often look dull and uneven. And the lifestyle choices you have made in the past are starting to show – excessive exposure to sun, smoke, stress, poor diet and dehydration will cause your skin to lose its collagen, glow and elasticity.

There are many factors that contribute to premature aging. Sitting in front of computers for hours on end, drinking copious amounts of coffee, snacking on sugary foods and living with high stress levels all attack the skin from the inside out. Then there are the outside elements such as central heating, sun exposure and atmospheric pollution. Whilst you cannot avoid all of these, you certainly can live with awareness and reduce your exposure as much as possible.

Your skin mirrors your lifestyle choice; the way it looks has less to do with your age than how it has been treated. Only 20 percent of lines are certain, the rest is down to the way you live your life. The positive news is that skin renews itself every 21 days - you just need to encourage it a little.

It is much easier to prevent damage than try to repair it, however there are ways to put the brakes on premature aging and get your skin back to a radiant glow.

- Stop smoking, after sun damage smoking is the biggest cause of premature aging. This happens due to the nicotine constricting your blood vessels and decreasing the flow of oxygen to your skin.

- Use a retinoid cream every day or every couple of days. Dermatologists claim that a daily application of a prescription retinoid lotion can erase years from your skin.
- Renew and boost your skin with a weekly facial. There is no need for expensive salon visits you can easily do a DIY facial at home which will be just as effective. Block out 30 minutes in your calendar each week to give yourself a facial – make sure you include a cleanse, exfoliate, mask, face steam and finish off with a nourishing face moisturizer.
- Rain, hail or shine – make sure that you wear a sunscreen every day. It takes as little as 20 minutes of unprotected sun exposure to damage your skin.
- Take time to relax and get a natural facelift. Stress wreaks havoc with your hormones, which can damage your skin. By taking the time to chill out your face muscles will relax and you will look much more soft and serene.
- Nourish and hydrate your skin with a daily moisturizer. Moisturizing will plump out the fine lines to give you a radiant glow. Look for moisturizers that have age-fighting ingredients like vitamin A (retinols), kinetin or vitamin C. Remember to not neglect your neck and chest as these are one of the first areas to show signs of aging.
- Don't tan. Tanning causes wrinkles and age spots. Even if wrinkles haven't shown up yet, you need to stop tanning now because you can be sure that they will show up in the future. If you do have sun damage? You can reverse the damage with photo rejuvenation such as pulsed light treatments or micro-dermabrasion.

- Cleanse your face every night. This helps remove all the toxins and impurities that have got caught in your skin throughout the day. All the smoke, traffic fumes and pollution that you are exposed to everyday. If the residue is not cleansed away then it can do damage to your skin.
- Eat a diet high in essential fats and antioxidants. These foods help repair the damage of premature aging by restoring and rebuilding strong skin cells. Eat plenty of raw nuts, avocadoes, salmon, blueberries, mangos and vegetable oils.
- Delay the aging process with clean living. Breathe in some fresh country air, eat a diet rich in wholefoods and find time to relax.
- Exfoliate three times a week to leave you fresh faced. By removing the older layers of the skin, you encourage cell renewal. It is the new cells that keep your skin looking bright and vibrant.

For a little herbal infusion try the Parsley Toner. *Use for normal/ dry skins. Chop 1/2 cup of parsley and cover it with 1 cup boiling water. After it cools, strain and store it in a jar. Apply using a cotton ball. You can also store in a spritzer bottle.*

11. Purify With a Clay Mask

Clay masks are a must. They naturally draw out any impurities and toxins from the skin when applied, leaving the skin feeling supple and fresh. When applied, the high mineral content of clay rejuvenates the skin and naturally draws out any impurities and toxins. The earthiness of the clay exfoliates and polishes the skin, removing dead skin cells and buildup in the pores to bring about a smooth healthy glow.

There are various clays used in beauty masks – all offering different healing properties. Below are a few popular clays:

1. **Rose Clay** is mild kaolin clay that can be used on normal to dry skin to gently cleanse and exfoliate the skin while improving the skin's circulation. Rose Clay is tinted with iron oxides and is often used to give a beautiful pink color to soaps and powders.
2. **White Kaolin Clay** is the mildest of all clays. White Kaolin Clay is suitable for sensitive skin. It helps stimulate circulation to the skin while gently exfoliating and cleansing it. White Kaolin Clay does not draw oils from the skin and can be used on dry skin types.
3. **French Green Clay** is the most commonly used therapeutic clay. French Green Clay is rich in minerals and phyto-nutrients and often used in day spas for facials and body wraps. French Green Clay is highly effective at drawing oils and toxins out from the skin. This clay is not recommended for dry or sensitive skin.

Although there are many wonderful properties and benefits of clay masks, be careful if you have dry or sensitive skin. Always do a patch test on your skin and talk to a professional if you are unsure.

Try the French Green Clay Facial Mask (great for acne prone skin)

- 4 Tablespoons French Green Clay
- 5 dried bay leaves

- 1 cup distilled water

Boil one cup of water and add bay leaves. Slowly add the liquid to the clay to form a thick paste. Apply to face and allow to dry. Leave on for 15 to 20 minutes then rinse with warm water

For a little holistic bliss try these face Scrubs from nature - 100% natural

Chia seed scrub

- *1 tsp. chia seeds*
- *1 tsp. almond meal*
- *1 tbsp. almond oil*

Mix together. Scrub over face and neck and leave for 10 minutes.

Oats and yogurt scrub

- *1 tbsp. rolled oats*
- *1 tbsp. natural yogurt*

Mix together. Scrub over face and neck and leave for 10 minutes.

12. Access Your Skin

Knowledge is power, and knowing your own skin type will help you understand exactly what your skin needs. The cosmetic industry likes to label you and your skin, and it can often get overwhelming when choosing a product. Take a few moments now to access your skin type so that you can treat it accordingly. Remember to do regular assessments as your skin changes throughout the years.

How does your skin look? Be honest. Look closely at it in the daylight; examine each pore and fine line. Touch it – is it smooth and even? Pull your cheeks – do they spring back quickly? Do you have dark circles or clogged pores?

Sensitive skin is easily irritated by perfumes and active skincare ingredients. The best way to know if you have sensitive skin is to access whether you get itchy or red after using a product. If you do – then you have sensitive skin. You need to use fragrance and alcohol free products and try to stick to completely natural products instead.

Dry skin feels tight and flaky. It develops fine lines and early wrinkles. If you have dry skin you need to ensure that you protect it against the elements. Avoid harsh and drying products that contain alcohol and soap. Use a night serum for a hydration and nutrition boost.

Normal skin is near perfect. It is soft and poreless. It doesn't dry, flake or become oily. It is hard to maintain normal skin – drink plenty of water and cleanse your face twice daily.

Combination skin is the most common type. The classic T-zone – forehead, nose and chin – is shiny and has clogged pores. While the skin around the eyes, cheeks and neck is dry. Use products designed for combination skin and do an intensive face scrub on your T-zone once a week.

Oily skin looks shiny and is prone to spots and blemishes. The skin produces more oil and has a thicker texture and is more likely to have clogged pores and blackheads. Gentle cleansing is paramount. Over-zealous scrubbing stimulates the oil glands to produce more oil. Choose mild and gentle cleansers and ensure you do a steam clean once a week.

An antiseptic from nature. *Tea tree oil has a long history of medicinal use and has been successful in treating acne, psoriasis and eczema. Simply place a few drops of tea tree oil on a cotton swab and apply it to the affected area of your skin. Be careful not to use too much, or you could end up drying your skin out. Avoid using tea tree oil if you are already using a product benzoyl peroxide.*

13. The Perfect Face Kit

Here is a list of things you need in your cosmetic drawer to keep a flawless face.

- **A good cleanser**- choose one that works with your skin type. Olive oil and coconut oil work for all skin types and are a great natural alternative.

- **A nourishing day cream** - moisturizers range from a basic day cream to an active antioxidant anti-aging cream – look for creams with sun protection. The purpose of a day cream is to act as a barrier to the skin and keep the moisture locked in. Rich, textured creams suit normal, dry and mature skins. Light lotions are ideal for normal or sensitive skins. Oil free creams are recommended for combination or oily skin tones.

- **Night cream** – night creams will feed your skin whilst you sleep. Look for a nourishing, rich cream that will give your skin a delicious boost. If you find that your skin gets congested after using a night cream – then it is probably best that you do not apply. If you are over 35 and have damaged skin you may opt for an advanced anti-aging cream. These are filled with active ingredients such as retinol and AHAs.

- **Eye products** – eye products are not an indulgence, they are essential. They are designed to repair and nourish fine lines and crepe like skin.

- **Sun protection** – sun protection is the most effective anti-aging product that you can use.

- **Lip balm** – invest in a nourishing lip balm to apply every few hours. This will keep your lips delicate and smooth.
- **Good mirror** – you need to be able to view your skin well. Invest in a good magnetic mirror. Check regularly for clean pores, dry patches and fine lines.
- **Facial exfoliator** – this product is what makes the difference between good skin and great skin. Use twice a week to buff and polish the skin.

"Some people, no matter how old they get, never lose their beauty - they merely move it from their faces into their hearts." ~ Martin Buxbaum

14. Looking After Your Lips

After your eyes, your lips are the most vulnerable area in the fight against ageing. Unlike your face, the skin that makes up your lips is much more delicate and finer – which makes them much more exposed to ageing. Some ways that you can treat your lips right are:

- Drink plenty of water to keep your lips hydrated and plump.

- Don't wait for your lips to become dry and cracked, use an intensive lip balm for nourishment and hydration every few hours.

- Apply a conditioning mask to your lips while you sleep. Mix 5ml of vitamin E oil with one drop of rose essential oil. Apply at night and leave on. This treatment will give your lips an instant shine.

15. Exfoliate

There are few beauty treatments that deliver instant results like a face scrub. Exfoliation is the key to glowing skin because it removes dull, dead cells from the skins surface to expose the fresher and brighter skin beneath.

You should exfoliate once a week after you have cleansed your face, using either a grainy scrub, buffing cloth or a chemical exfoliant.

- **Buffing clothes** – these are the most gentle way to buff the skin to a radiant polish. You can either buy a buffing clothe from your local beauty store, otherwise a cotton face clothe will do the job just fine. To exfoliate your face, wet the cloth with warm water, wring it out and gently press into your skin for a count of 10. Wipe away any residue and repeat 2-3 times.
- **Grainy scrubs** – these scrubs contain tiny particles which when massaged into your skin help to lift out impurities and remove old skin. You can make your

own holistic and natural scrubs at home which are just as effective as their expensive counterparts.

<blockquote>
<u>For oil and combination skin try a lemon and sugar scrub.</u>

Mix a handful of brown sugar with the juice of half a lemon. Massage gently into your skin, not forgetting about your chest. Wipe off with a damp cotton cloth. Rinse thoroughly with warm water and pat dry. Apply a nourishing face cream.

<u>For normal to dry skin try a peachy scrub</u>

Pulp one large peach and mix with one tablespoon of ground oatmeal. Massage over your face paying extra attention to congested areas. Wipe off with a damp cotton cloth. Rinse thoroughly with warm water and pat dry. Apply a nourishing face cream.
</blockquote>

- **Chemical exfoliators** – These exfoliants contain the active ingredients of enzymes and AHAs. These exfoliants work by dissolving dead skin cells, leaving the skin brighter and smoother.

16. Anti-Ageing Facial Massage

A quick pressure-point massage relieves tension and aids lymphatic drainage. A face massage will give an instant lift and youthful look to your face. Master the technique of face massage and you will boost the tone and texture of your complexion.

The benefits of a face massage are endless:

- It will leave your skin nourished and glowing. Steady rhythmic pressure to the face gets the blood flowing to the surface of the skin, which then nourishes the skin with goodness.
- A gentle face massage will leave your skin bright and fresh. The gentle pressure helps to remove any dead skin cells, turning dull complexions into a glowing beauty.
- Massage warms up your skin, making it ideal for your skin to soak up all the goodness from any oils and creams you put on.

17. Tiny Red Thread Veins

The little red veins that are found more commonly on the cheeks and nose of fair skinned people are caused by exposure to heat, cold or wind. Make sure you treat your skin gently to combat these little red veins. Avoid using very hot water and protect your skin in extreme temperatures. Wear a moisturizer daily, and an SPF 15 sunscreen to prevent any further damage.

18. Treat Acne

There is nothing worse than a persistent case of acne that you cannot get rid of. Along with your treatment plan from your dermatologist try a few of these holistic remedies that may have your skin clearing up in no time.

- **Get more Zinc**. Either take supplements or eat more foods rich in zinc. Zinc helps to fight the bacterium that causes acne. A diet low in zinc can actually cause acne breakouts.
- **Sweeten up with honey** – try a honey mask 1-2 times per week. Honey is loaded with antibacterial properties so it is great for disinfecting and healing acne breakouts. Simply apply raw honey to your face and let it sit for 20 minutes. Rinse off with warm water and pat dry.
- **Wash your face twice a day**. Help remove the impurities by washing them down the drain. Make sure that you are gentle, as over scrubbing can

stimulate your sebaceous glands to produce more sebum, which will lead to increasing your acne.

- **Take a high grade multi-vitamin** - Acne is often a reflection that your body is not in balance. Your skin needs good nutrition to give it the energy to repair and restore skin. Try taking a chromium supplement once a day to promote healing and future breakouts.

Beauty Tip: *Carry a bottle of facial mist in your handbag so that you can spritz and refresh your face throughout the day. It is great for spraying before applying moisturizers to help increase hydration. And it works wonders when spritzed over your make up to help lock it in for the day. Keep a bottle in your bag, at your desk, by your bed and don't fly without it.*

19. Load up on antioxidants

It has been proven that the antioxidants found in wine, tea, chocolate, blueberries, grapes, and other fruits and vegetables can help prevent aging and increase your wellness. As you age, the repair of your cells slow down, however this can be improved by getting an adequate supply of antioxidants. In short, antioxidants load up the cells with a boost of energy and goodness so that they can repair more quickly. Overall this helps slow down the effects of aging.

As a general rule, the richer the color of the fruit or vegetable, the more antioxidants it contains. For radiant and youthful skin start sipping on green tea and savor salmon, blueberries, mangos and any fruit or vegetable that is brightly colored.

20. Hydrate And Look Younger

At the age of 49 a youthful Demi Moore reminds us *"I moisturize, moisturize, moisturize. No matter how late it is, when I get home, I take the time to clean and moisturize my face. I'm a big believer in that if you focus on good skin care, you really won't need a lot of makeup."* Hydration is the key to flawless skin and timeless beauty, the water plumps up the skin which decreases fine lines and wrinkles. To keep your body well hydrated use a hydrating face cream and drink at least two liters of water a day.

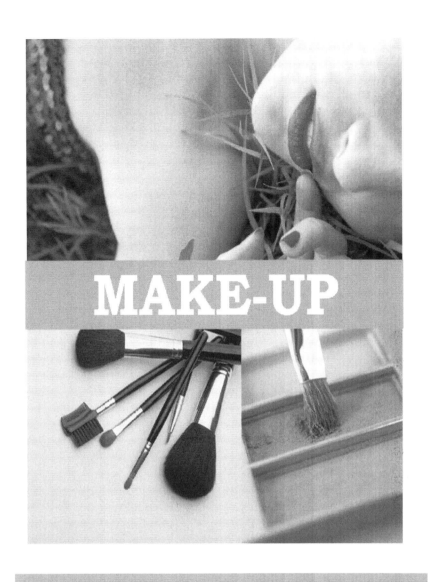

Beauty Tip: Learn to accept your flaws and embrace them. For it is the quirky things that make you authentic and beautiful

21. Kissable Lips

Did you know that your lips are most balanced when the upper and lower lips are equal in size or thickness?

Make lips look fuller: Full lips are really fashionable and if you want to make your lips look fuller, then simply apply a lip pencil just outside the natural lip line. Choose bright and bold colors and finish off the look by applying a glossy lip lacquer over top.

Make lips look smaller: If you want to make your lips look smaller then draw the lip pencil just inside the natural lip line, and choose colors that are close to your natural lip color.

For more youthful looking lips: For mature lips choose lighter lipsticks that do not have too much color. More natural and earthy tones work best. Remember to hydrate and nourish your lips every couple of hours with a lip balm.

For uneven lips: If you have uneven lips and one side of the natural bow is larger than the other then a decision needs to be made on whether to make your lips larger or smaller - in order to even out the lip shape. Simply use a lip pencil to redefine and fill out uneven lips.

22. The Secrets Of Concealer

When using concealer ensure that you use one shade lighter than your foundation to cover up the dark shadowy areas around your eyes. If you use one that is too light, you will emphasize the darkness, making it look quite blue. However if you are trying to hide imperfections on the skin, use a concealer that is the same color as your skin.

Many makeup artists prefer to use concealer on its own so that skin looks fresh and natural.

How to apply concealer

Beauty Tip: Always use a fine brush when applying concealer.

Dark Circles – to hide dark circles hold a mirror at eye level, look ahead and then tilt your chin downwards to show the dark circles at its worst. Carefully paint the concealer onto the dark areas only, patting lightly into place.

Bags under the eyes – Apply the concealer on the area of shadow directly beneath the bags, not on the bags themselves – otherwise you will highlight your bags.

23. The Magic of Light Reflecting Highlighting Crème

Illuminating crème's are a great way to add some highlight to your cheeks, eyelids, brow bones or lips. They can create a natural and dewy look, one that will leave you looking radiant and fresh. Illuminating makeup is also great for reducing the appearance of fine lines, as the light weight consistency does not get molded in wrinkles and the light reflecting properties distract from your fine lines.

Beauty Tip: For a more lightweight foundation, dilute your current foundation with some face cream. Perfectly light and sheer for the warmer months.

24. Fix Your Face Shape

Most of us were not blessed with perfect bone structure and there is bound to be something that you wish you could change. With a little skill and practice you can change the features of your face with a subtle approach – it is called 'Contouring'. Contouring is the art of highlighting and shading. It is where you simply use a highlight color one or two shades lighter than your skin tone to make an area more prominent and anything darker than your skin tone will make that area recede.

Before you get started it is important to study your bone structure with your hair pulled back off your face. Decide which area or feature you would like to alter, keeping in mind that light projects and dark recedes.

Here's how you can easily alter your face:

To Contour - Use a bronzing powder a shade or two darker than your skin tone

To Highlight – Use a highlighting powder one to two shades lighter than your skin tone. (You can also use blush to highlight your cheek bones)

Refer to diagram

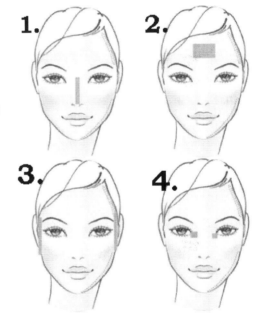

1. **Contour –**
   Pushes back a
   protruding nose
   Highlight –
   Brings a flat
   nose forward.
   Slims a wide
   nose or
   elongates a
   short nose.

2. **Contour** – Flattens a protruding forehead
   Highlight – Brings forward an indented forehead,
   enlarges forehead.

3. **Contour** – Slims a wide face.
   Highlight – Widens a narrow face

4. **Contour** – Brings wide set eyes closer together

Highlight – Gives the illusion that close set eyes are wider apart.

Beauty Tip: If you want to look a little more awake use a cream colored pencil on the inside of your eye, it opens up your eyes and makes them pop.

25. The Secrets To Wearing Red Lipstick

Re-invent yourself with a little burst of color. Color has the power to uplift and energize you – this applies to lipstick also. Wearing red lipstick is empowering, it creates a sense of energy, strength, passion and seduction. It will give you an instant boost on those days that you feel sluggish. There is a red lipstick for every skin tone. Here is a basic guide to picking the right lipstick:

- **Orange based red lipsticks for warmer skin tones** –A warmer skin tone has a golden or more yellow undertone and typically looks great in gold jewelry. If you tan when out in the sun then you have a warm skin tone. Another way to determine is to look at your veins and they should have a greener cast to them.
- **Red lipstick with blue undertones suit cooler skin tones** - Note that you can have a cool skin tone even if you have darker skin. A sure fire way to figure out if you are a cooler skin tone is if you look good in silver

jewelry. Again look at your veins and if they have a bluish cast, you are a cool skin tone.

Now that you have dared to purchase your red lipstick, can you not help but wonder how some women apply it so perfect – they look impeccable and stylish with their perfect red lips? You can't help but wonder "how do they not get it everywhere"? Well wonder no more – here are some insider tricks to keeping your red lipstick looking flawless all day long.

- First line well moisturized lips with a red lip pencil. Take care to get the shape perfect. Now color the entire lip in with the lip pencil.
- After you have carefully painted on your first coat of red lipstick, blot it with a tissue. Brush a light dusting of face powder over your lips and press the tissue onto your lips.
- Apply a second coat of red lipstick with care and precision. Blot again with the tissue.
- If you want a glossy finish, simply add a little bit of clear lip glass over the top.

26. Perfect Lashes

Your eyes are the window to your soul – you need them to stand out. Here is a sure fire way to get lashes that make a statement – follow these directions to give the illusion of bigger and more dramatic eyes.

First you always have to curl your lashes before applying your mascara. To curl your lashes simply look straight ahead into the mirror and position the curlers around the upper lashes, ensuring that you do not catch any skin. Press down firmly for a count of 10. Then roll the curler upwards and away while still gripping the lashes. Release and repeat on the other eye.

Now it is time to add some oomph with mascara. It is best to use two different types of mascara – for example have volumising mascara and lengthening mascara. Coat the lashes with the first mascara and then do a second coat in the alternate mascara. Keep building up coats until you have the desired length and volume.

Beauty Tip: Want to make your small eyes look bigger? Stay away from dark eye shadows. Start with a nude base, and then apply an eye shadow a color or two darker than the base shadow. Use your finger to blend the color up toward your eyebrow.

27. Choose Your Focus

When applying strong makeup (like smoky eyes or red lips) put the focus on either eyes or lips - never both. If you decide to play up your eyes then make sure you stick with a nearly nude lipstick to balance out the look. Or counter a bold lip statement with a sheer wash of beige or caramel eye shadow and mascara.

28. Line And Define Your Eyes

Eye liner is a women's best friend, the definition makes the eyes look alluring. There are several techniques you can use when applying eyeliner, make sure you choose the one to best suit your eye shape.

A little eyeliner placed on the outer corners of your lower lids will highlight your eyes and make them appear larger. Unless you have large eyes, refrain from applying dark eyeliners inside your lids, as they will make your eyes look smaller. When you apply eyeliner to the top and bottom lid, make sure that they meet at the outer corner.

For a discreet daytime eyeliner, apply a little eyeliner on the underside of the lower lashes only.

A handy hint: Line the inside of eyes with a white eye pencil to make them look more bright and awake.

Eye liners do not have to come in a pencil form. Makeup experts often use eye shadows to make up some of the best crowd stopping eyeliners. For a deep and precise line take an eyeliner brush, wet it, then dab the wet brush into the pot of eye shadow. Glide the eye shadow along the lash line. You can also use eye shadows without wetting the eyeliner brush first. Either way, eyeliner is necessary for a lush lash look.

Beauty Tip: Trying to look well rested when you aren't? Avoid piling on the foundation. Use a tinted moisturizer and line your eyes with a beige eye pencil — it counteracts any redness around your eyes.

Beauty Wisdom *"For attractive lips, speak words of kindness"* – Audrey Hepburn

29. Be Cheeky

Blusher gives your face a vibrant lift. Don't waste your time trying to contour high cheekbones when there is none to begin with. You will only end up with a bad 1980's makeup job. All makeup artists agree that blush looks best when applied to the apple of the cheek – this is where color would normally rush to if you were embarrassed or flushed.

The apple is the round, lifted part of your cheek when you smile. To apply the blush simply smile and dust on some blush in a circular motion. Make sure that you blend the color in with your hairline at the sides. Blush should always be the final step of your make-up routine.

Some Blushing rules

- Find a blush color that makes you look healthy and natural.
- A blush should blend naturally – if you have to work extra hard to blend it in, then it is to dark or too bright.
- Own two different shades of blush: one that gives you a healthy and natural glow and one that is a little brighter for a pop of color.
- Be bold and brave – try using your lipstick on your cheeks as you would a cream blush.

Beauty Tip: Take your blush from daytime to evening by sweeping on a brighter shade of blush and blending it slightly higher up on your cheekbones.

30. Drama With Color

When it comes to choosing the right colors to use on your eyes, you should always remember that opposites work best. If you use an opposite color eye shadow to the color of your eyes – your eyes will 'pop'. Look at a color wheel and choose the colors that are directly opposite your eye color. Remember this simple trick for when you need to buy your next eye shadow or eye pencil. Here's a cheat sheet:

For blue eyes: Orange is the opposite color of blue, choose colors with orange undertones like gold, apricot, or peach.

For green eyes: Red is the opposite color of green, choose colors that have red undertones, like deep plums, purples and wine.

For brown eyes: Brown is a neutral color, so any color will work well. For a little drama blues and purples look fantastic with brown eyes.

Beauty Tip: Turn back time - look younger with sheer and natural shades.

31. Maximize Your Eye Shape

- **Deep-Set Eyes** - Rely on pale, shimmery shades to enhance your eyes. Sweep a light shade across the top lid only, from the inner corner to just beyond the outer corner.

- **Wide-Set Eyes** - Create closeness by applying a deep shadow shade from the inner corner to mid-lid. Then apply a lighter shade from mid-lid to outer corner and blend where shades meet.

- **Close-Set Eyes** - Help them appear wider by applying a pale shade from the inner corner to mid-lid. Then apply a slightly deeper shade from mid-lid to outer corner and blend where shades meet.

- **When Wearing Glasses** - Forget about adding more color with eye shadows. Instead play up lashes with volumising black mascara. Take time to shape and define your eye brows—remember, brows should frame your eyes, not your frames.

- **Asian Eyes** - To bring out their beauty, create a thick, smoky line along top lashes—thick enough to be seen when your eye is open—and a thinner one under bottom lashes.

Beauty Tip: Refresh your makeup by spraying your face with water. While your face is still wet, start re-blending the foundation, powder, or concealer you already have on.

32. Create A Flawless Base

The purpose of foundation is to even out your skin tone, not to change the color of your skin or hide fine lines. You want a foundation that matches your face color exactly – so there is no point testing foundation on your wrists or the back of your hand. You need to check the color by applying a small test on your cheek, making sure that you always check the color in natural light.

When buying foundation, take your time to get the exact color, it is the most important part of your makeup.

Now that you have found the perfect color, applying the foundation should be extremely easy. Before you apply your foundation make sure you prime your face first – this will set the foundation and help keep your makeup flawless for a much longer time. When you are applying your foundation, remember less is more – only cover what you need – and there is no need to cover your neck. If you want a light and dewy coverage try applying the foundation with a damp makeup sponge. If you are seeking more coverage then apply your foundation with a brush.

Finish off your base with a brush of powder. This will set your foundation and make a perfect canvas for the rest of your makeup.

Goddess Style: Dust some gold eye shadow across your eyelids for a little radiance.

33. A Glowing 10 Minute Beauty

Some days you just don't feel like putting on a full face of makeup - try this quick ten minute makeup to get you looking good, without being to overdone.

- Cleanse and moisturize your skin
- Apply concealer under your eyes
- Blend in some foundation
- Powder over your face to set the base
- Fill in and shade eyebrows with an eye shadow or brow pencil
- Apply a light shade over your eyelid – a matte white is great for a fresh look

- Use a dark brown eye shadow to line your eyes and then apply one coat of mascara
- Brush a little blush or bronzer on your cheeks
- Perfect your pout with a lip stain or gloss

Beauty Tip: For stylish simplicity paint your nails red, tie your hair back into a sleek ponytail and do either a smoky eye or bold lips.

34. Beauty Tips For Your Hot Date

Before you leave home to go on a hot date with who could be Mr. Right, make sure have paid attention to the little details.

- Carry a tube of clear lip-gloss to add a sexy shine to lips – also looks great when applied to either the eyelids or cheekbones for a little natural gloss.
- Dust your chest, arms, back and legs with a shimmer highlight powder for a little evening glamour
- For a little subtle sexiness, apply a 3-4 single false eyelashes to the outside corner of each eye.
- Maximize your smile by brushing your teeth with a tooth-brightening toothpaste.

35. Soften Your Look

Go for a more natural and soft look by choosing to use brown mascara instead of black. And when you have lined your eyes, gently smudge the line with a brush for a soft and natural line. Try a light weight light reflecting foundation for a subtle glow and a dab of clear lip gloss to the lips for a healthy shine.

Often blacks and other dark shades can look harsh on the face. Try a softer look for a more flattering daytime look. The softness can often be more flattering, especially on mature women.

Beauty Tip: Narrow a broad nose by running a line of highlight powder or lighter foundation down the center of it. A broad nose may also be made finer by shading the sides with a darker foundation or a brushing of bronzer.

36. DE clutter Your Makeup Bag

Create less stress and more inner calm by simplifying and DE cluttering your makeup bag. As women we tend to over buy beauty products. Work out what you use regularly and just keep that in your make-up bag. Store your other beauty products that you don't use on a daily basis in a makeup case. Remember to toss out any old makeup, or makeup that has leaked. While you have all your makeup out, wipe over all the cases and replace all your old sponges. Now is also a great time to clean and sterilize your makeup brushes – soak them in a little bit of tea tree oil mixed with water.

Make up does not last forever – here is a guide to your makeup's life span:

- Foundation – 12-18 months
- Concealer – 1 year
- Powder – 2 years
- Mascara – 3-6 months
- Lipstick – 12-18 months
- Lip or eye pencil – 1 year
- Eye shadow – 1 year
- Powder blush – 2 years
- Cream blush – 6 months – 1 year
- Moisturizer -12-18 months
- Eye cream – 1 year
- SPF lotion – 1 year

Beauty Tip: Widen close-set eyes by creating the illusion of a greater space between your eyebrows. Pluck you eyebrows to widen the gap between both your eyebrows.

37. Melt Down Your Lipsticks

Most women have an overflowing drawer of lipsticks that they hardly wear – this often causes overwhelm. A great handy tip to organize your lipsticks is to melt them down. Purchase a small thimble container and melt down your lipsticks into the thimble bases. To melt down your lipstick simply put it in a glass bowl and set it in a saucepan of boiling water – once melted pour the lipstick into the thimble base and allow it to cool and set.

You now have a variety of lipstick colors all neatly organized. Apply the lipstick with a retractable lipstick brush – and don't forget to apply the lip liner first.

38. The Perfect Brow

Fill in your brow for a little subtle emphasis – this is one of the greatest beauty secrets of makeup artists. Using a brow pencil or eye shadow that complements your natural shade fill in your brows like so:

- Begin at the inner corner of the eyebrow. Fill in color with tiny, upward, feathery strokes, working in the direction of hair growth.
- Give an extra lift to the brow by applying some color along the upper edge of the brow to accentuate the arch.
- For a little more drama subtly extent the line at the outer ends.

39. Revamp And Reinvent

Have a little fun and get creative with makeup and try different looks – don't get stuck in the rut of wearing the same makeup for over a decade. Every month try something new. Read magazines and books for inspiration and even visit your local department store for a free makeup lesson. Most importantly don't be a slave to fashion and the latest trends – stick with techniques that suit you.

> **Beauty Tip:** For a little drama give your face a color boost. Try navy, purple or yellow mascara. It's a great way to be a little daring and have a little fun.

40. Embrace Your Age

As you get older you naturally develop lines. Don't try to hide them by caking on half a bottle of foundation; it only draws attention to them. Lines are the map to your face, they show your character, choose to own and embrace them. Here are some ways to wear your makeup that will flatter your lines and boost your radiant:

- Moisture skin well before applying makeup.
- Use cream formulas for your concealers and foundations as they are less likely to get caked in lines. Try to find ones with light reflection properties.
- Keep your lips well moisturized and nourished, this will reduce the appearance of fine lines in that area. Choose creamy lipsticks and a matching lip liner to keep the color from bleeding into the lines.

- Avoid all shimmer eye shadows, for they work their way into creases and accentuate any fine lines you have on your eyelids.
- Use a lip liner for volume and definition. As we age we lose definition in our lips – give them a boost with a little lip liner.
- Keep happy thoughts. The more happy and content you are the more relaxed and wrinkle free your face will be.
- Pencil in and define your eyebrows for an instant face lift.
- Wear a dusting of bronzer for a healthy and youthful glow.
- Try a brown or grey mascara as opposed to black. Black can be more harsh and aging on mature skins

Beauty Wisdom: *"Nobody grows old merely by living a number of years. We grow old by deserting our ideals. Years may wrinkle the skin, but to give up enthusiasm wrinkles the soul. "~* Samuel Ullman

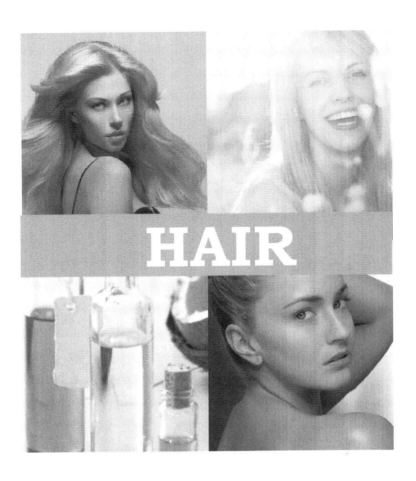

41. Foods For Glossy Hair

What you eat plays a significant role in determining the health of your hair and scalp. A diet rich in protein is vital for healthy hair. If you want to improve the strength and natural shine of your hair, then step up your intake of fish, seaweed, almonds, brazil nuts, yogurt and coconut oil.

Eat lots of lean meat, eggs, nuts, seeds, and pulses, carrots, and greens. And Cut down on caffeine and alcohol, for these stimulants hamper the absorption of minerals essential for hair health.

Beauty Tip: Give yourself a regular head massage, it stimulates your circulation and nourishes your hair and scalp.

42. A Coconut Nourishing Hair Mask

Bring a little tropical infusion into your home – try a coconut hair mask. Coconut oil is widely used in the pacific islands and islander women can thank the natural benefits of coconut oil for their long, healthy tresses.

If you have dry, damaged hair from excessive coloring, perming, or styling, then this treatment will restore your hair back to how it should look – thicker, shinier and lustrous.

Coconut oil is a fantastic remedy for scalp problems like dryness, itchiness and dandruff. Coconut oil is jam packed with goodness like calcium, iron, magnesium, and potassium. It also contains lauric acid, which has antifungal and antimicrobial properties, as well as moisturizing and calming benefits.

All you have to do is apply some coconut oil to your hair and massage it through. Leave it on overnight so that the oil can feed your hair with all its tropical goodness. Make sure that you wear a shower cap to bed and be sure to lay an extra towel over your pillowcase. In the morning wash and style your hair as normal.

After just one treatment you will be blessed with glossier and smoother locks. If you are suffering from dandruff this treatment works miracles at getting rid of it. Also another tip – if your ends are a little dry, split and brittle, apply a small amount of coconut oil to the very ends, and style as usual. This treatment is a gift from nature and it will leave your hair thanking you.

43. Embrace Your Natural style

Women everywhere are covering up their natural hair – they are straightening their curls, coloring over their natural color and trying to achieve the opposite of what nature blessed them with.

Every day we are bombarded with beauty advice as magazines, billboards and products tell us what is beautiful. The secret of beauty is not in the latest hair product or expensive haircut. The secret of beauty is embracing your own natural style whilst enhancing it subtly with products and trends. The truth is that nature knows best – and what you were given naturally is what will work best for you.

Natural is beautiful and nothing in nature is ever copied - it's unique.

Learning how to embrace your natural style whether it is with your hair, your life or with your clothes, will set you one your own authentic path, it will free your soul and make you radiate with a deep natural beauty that cannot be purchased or copied.

Beauty Tip: Nourish your hair with Argon Oil, and then put it up in a bun with the product in. After a few hours take it out of the bun and you will have glossy beach waves.

44. Nourish Your Hair

Beautiful and shiny hair is a reflection of perfect health. Healthy hair makes you look healthy, vibrant and radiant. To treat your hair well you want to ensure that it is receiving all the vitamins that it needs to repair.

Bottom line is that when your body is nourished, so is your hair. Nourish your hair from the inside out. Eat a diet high in wholefoods and take a vitamin C supplement with a high grade multi vitamin every day.

If you want an extra boost for your hair then look at investing in a hair vitamin supplement from your local pharmacy. Look for supplements that contain a rich source of B complex, iron, zinc, biotin, folic acid, flax seed oil, silica and/or pantothenic acid.

Beauty Tip: Add more luster, warmth and richness to your hair – get some gold, honey, caramel or red highlights.

45. Scalp Massage

A simple scalp massage for 5 minutes a day can give you thicker, healthier and glossier hair. It also helps your hair grow faster. Massage stimulates your circulation which then brings a rich supply of blood to your scalp. Your blood brings nutrients to the hair follicles, feeding your hair with nourishment and goodness. The better flow of blood circulation to your scalp the healthier your hair will be.

When you massage your scalp you can either do it dry or wet. You may want to consider massaging an oil like coconut oil or olive oil into your scalp for a holistic treatment. Or you could make up your own blissful treatment. Mix up 40 drops each of rosemary, lavender, thyme and lemon oil into a 100ml bottle of pure almond oil. This is a lovely light fragrant massage oil that brings the spa to your home.

The Technique: When you massage your scalp ensure that you use the pads of your fingers. Spread your fingers apart and place them firmly on your head. Move in little circles starting at the base of your neck and slowly working your way up to your forehead. Not only will this treatment nourish your hair, it will distress you and leave you feeling invigorated and refreshed.

If you're short on time you can massage your scalp while you wash your hair

46. For A Burst Of Growth

If you want your hair to grow quicker, then, you need to ensure you get a haircut every 6-8 weeks. Your ends are the oldest and driest part of your hair, they are likely to split and damage your hair if you do not get them regularly trimmed.

No matter how gentle you are to your hair, the ends split and move farther up the hair shaft, causing tangles, which then lead to breakage and snapping. The only way to avoid this is to get a regular trim.

Beauty Tip: Like your skin, you need to feed your hair, from the inside out...and the outside in.

47. Become A Natural Beauty

You are doing your hair and body a huge favor if you reduce the chemicals you put in your body - and that includes what you put on your body and hair. When your body has to spend time breaking down toxins it has no time to repair other areas of your body such as hair, nails and skin. It has to prioritize where it spends its energy and unfortunately beautifying the body is not a priority – disease fighting always takes priority.

To give your body a little boost, free up some of its energy by not making it have to work so hard. Give it a break from having to remove toxins and chemicals from your body by choosing natural and toxic free shampoos, conditioners, hairsprays and serums.

To bring life, shine and bounce back to distressed hair try a few DIY products. Here are a few holistic remedies to get you inspired:

- To tame the frizz try coconut oil as a hair treatment and serum.
- To gloss up your hair, try a rinse made with apple cider vinegar and water.
- To help your hair grow faster mix a little ylang ylang with almond oil and massage on to your scalp.

There are loads of natural alternatives for hair problems and concerns, get curious and start researching, you will be amazed at what you discover.

48. Let Your Hair Breathe

The elements can wreak havoc with your hair – things like the pollution, traffic fumes and smoke all leave residue in your hair. When your hair is filled with residue it is harder for your scalp to breathe and oxygenate. Your hair has difficulty in breathing and absorbing nutrients, and if the residue is not properly cleansed it will then prevent your hair from looking sleek and healthy.

To reduce the residue in your hair, wash your hair every second day and swap your shampoo and conditioner brand with another brand every two or three months. Vegetable oils are also great for deep cleansing – so try and do an intensive oil treatment once a week – try using coconut oil, olive oil or almond oil.

Beauty Tip: Before shampooing your hair, add olive oil to the ends. It will help give a deep cleanse along with being a fantastic detangler.

49. Straight Hair Is Shinier

Straightening your hair will make your hair look much shinier. The reason behind this madness is that more light is reflected off straight hair shafts as opposed to curly or wavy ones.

Give it a go and see for yourself – create a sleek and elegant straight style for the day. To create a sleek and straight style you need to start by putting a small amount of high quality hair serum through the ends of your hair to prevent heat damage and frizz. With your hair dryer gently dry your hair straight, using a radial brush to grip the hair - giving you maximum control.

The secret is to ensure that your hair cuticles are dried flat by keeping the hairdryer nozzle pointing downwards towards the end of the hair shaft at all times. Once your hair is dry, run a straightening iron through your hair to give you extra sleekness. Finish with a small amount of shine serum rubbed into only the ends of your hair.

Don't be over zealous with the hair drying or straightening – as you don't want to do any heat damage.

50. Become An Italian Beauty

Unlock the secrets of olive oil and follow what the Italian women have known for years - olive oil promotes beauty. The Mediterranean diet and lifestyle – rich in olive oil - is what helps so many Italian beauties glow from the inside out.

Italian woman have given themselves weekly head massages with olive oil for years. This intensive treatment helps repair split ends, heals dandruff, and makes your hair shiny, silky, and lustrous.

Massage a few tablespoons of olive oil into the scalp and hair. Cover your hair with a plastic shower cap and leave on for 30 minutes or more, then shampoo as usual. (it is a great idea to keep the shower caps that you get from hotels for this reason)

> **Beauty Tip:** Revive your hair by tipping your head upside down and spraying the roots with a volumizing spray. Allow 60 seconds to dry, and then bring your head back up.

51. Hair Repair

Your hair says so much about you; it is an expression of who you are. If you have glossy, healthy and stylish hair, it will make you look and feel fabulous, no matter what you're wearing.

Often we wreak havoc with our hair through over styling, overheating, over coloring and poor conditioning. When your hair is damaged it loses its luster, shine and brilliance. Here are some hair repair tips to revamp your damaged hair:

Treat Dandruff – Get out your juicer and pulp 2-3 apples. Apply the natural elixir onto your hair from the roots to the tips. Massage for 10 minutes and then shampoo and condition as normal. Massaging coconut oil into your hair is also great for treating dandruff.

Dry Hair Repair – The secret to repairing dry hair is hidden within the cupboards of your kitchen. Tame the frizz with this nourishing conditioner made from eggs and avocados.

Shampoo your hair first, and then feed your hair by massaging a mask of 1 beaten egg mixed well with 1 tsp. avocado oil. Let it sit for 10 minutes. Rinse well.

Detox your Hair- Get rid of the entire residue and junk that gets trapped in your hair every day. Purify your hair by massaging a paste made with bicarb soda and water. Massage into the roots, and then rinse out. Shampoo and condition as normal.

Treat Oily Hair – Before washing your hair with your regular shampoo, apply this pre-wash first. Mix 2 ripe bananas with 2 tbsp. of full-fat natural yogurt. Mash the bananas well and mix in the yogurt. Lather this mixture in your hair from the roots down, ensuring you work it through every inch. Cover with a shower cap and warm towel. Then relax for 20 minutes or longer. Rinse out with cool water. Then shampoo as per normal.

Beauty Tip: To curl the ends under, dry your hair and spray a radial brush with some hairspray. Roll the ends under the brush and heat with a hairdryer. Make sure you hit the cooling button to lock in the curl before unrolling.

52. A Sleek Ponytail

Knowing how to do a sleek ponytail will add class and elegance to every outfit – no matter if it with your jeans on a

Sunday morning or sipping cocktails with your girlfriends in your little black dress.

- Wash and shampoo your hair. Add some straightening serum and then dry your hair as normal.
- Run a straightening iron through your hair, section by section.
- For a little volume and height, backcomb the roots slightly at the crown of your head.
- Secure your ponytail with a hair tie and then wrap a small section of hair from underneath your ponytail around the hair tie. Fasten with a hair pin.
- Complete the look by applying a little shine serum or balm at the ends of the ponytail.

53. Lighter Hair Adds Youth

Most women over the age of 55 look too harsh with dark hair color – even if it is their natural color. This doesn't mean that you should go totally blonde as you get older, as that can look too severe as well. You just want to simply add a little warmth around your face by getting a few warm highlights. This will make you looker warmer, softer and more youthful.

Beauty Tip: Never brush wet hair, only run a wide toothed comb through it. Brushing wet hair will stretch hair beyond its elasticity, resulting in breaks and splits.

54. Enhance Your Curls

Make the most of what mother nature gave you and style your wavy hair into beachy and carefree. Dry your hair with a diffuser on the end of your hair dryer. Spray your hair with some sea salt mist and scrunch your hair. Repeat this process until your hair is dry and wavy. Make sure you set your hair dryer on a medium setting, as overheating dries out your hair and makes your curls fluffy. Don't brush your hair; just run your fingers through to detangle.

You can make your own sea salt mist by mixing 2 tbsp. of sea salt with 1 cup of boiling water. Stir until the salt has dissolved. Once cooled, put the solution in a spritz bottle.

55. A Salon Blow Wave

To get the perfect blow dry, use a round brush and dry your hair in sections. Start from the roots of the hair, running the brush and dryer all the way down to the end of the hair. Let that section of hair cool off for about five seconds, then repeat on another section. Alternating between heat and cool-down will give your hair more body and set your style.

For a little sex-kitten lift, after you have finished your blow-dry section off the hair on top of your head with some clips. Now divide that section into three parts and wrap a 2-inch Velcro hair roller around each section. Run your hair dryer over the rollers and finish with a gentle blast on the cold setting. Let your hair sit like this for 30 minutes, and then unwrap your strands, lightly brush them, and spray for hold.

Beauty Tip: Give Locks A Burst Of Cold. Before getting out of the shower turn the cold water on fully. Rinse your hair in cold water as it helps seal the cuticle, leaving you with a more sleek finish.

56. Blonde Ambition

If you want a natural looking blonde then try the latest trend "blondette" – think Kate Moss. This is the hair color du jour with modern city girls. This natural blonde is achieved by back-combing the ends of the hair to about half way up the hair shaft. The tips of the back-combing section are lightened, giving them a natural and sun-kissed look. To finish off the look the rest of the hair needs to be highlighted with a warm shade of blonde. This gives overall depth and tone.

Beauty Tip: Apply hair products 10 minutes before you style your hair. This helps your hair to fully absorb the product beforehand so that you get all of its benefits

57. Flatten Fly-Aways

There is nothing worse than putting in the time to blow-dry and create a beautiful sleek style, only to be destroyed by annoying fly- aways. No matter how much you spray your hair with hairspray they just will not sit flat. The best way to get them to sit flat is

- Start your style by spraying a little hairspray on your brush – as you brush your hair, your hair will become flat and smoother.
- Then if you still have persistent fly-aways – take a Kleenex tissue or paper towel and spray it with hairspray and wipe over your style.

58. Tousled Locks

A popular look which is super sexy is to have tousled locks that are straighter at the roots, with loose waves flowing from about 5-10cm from the roots. Think Sarah Jessica Parker.

To achieve this sexy tousled look:

- Wash and condition your hair.
- Put a curling serum in the ends.
- Wrap a terry cloth headband over the top of your head, flattening the roots of your hair.
- You can either blow dry your hair or leave it to dry naturally.
- When your hair is dried you will find that the headband has created a flat look on your roots.

- Gently lift the roots up with your fingers and lightly spray with hairspray.

Beauty Wisdom: *"Love of beauty is taste. The creation of beauty is art."* - Ralph Waldo Emerson

59. Protect Your Hair From The Sun

In summertime, we hear lots about protecting our skin from the sun but not so much about our hair. Excessive exposure to the sun can lead your hair to become faded, dry, brittle and lifeless. To protect your hair and stop unnecessary dehydration:

- Look for shampoos, conditioners and leave-in conditioners that offer UVA and UVB protection.
- Make your own SPF hair lotion. Simply dilute 2 teaspoons of SPF sun block with one cup of water. Using a spray bottle, spray the solution into damp hair before styling. For a boost of extra protection, you can mist the solution on throughout the day.

60. Hair Empowerment

Hair is your statement – it gives a little insight into who you are. And let's face it – when your hair looks great you feel wonderful. When you feel wonderful you are empowered to live life to the fullest and follow your dreams. A confident toss of the hair is very sexy – the world stops to admire. From today forward chose to own your beauty, because with a little effort and care for your hair, you will be able to create an uplifting feeling for yourself.

Beauty Wisdom: *"Taking joy in living is a woman's best cosmetic."* - Rosalind Russell

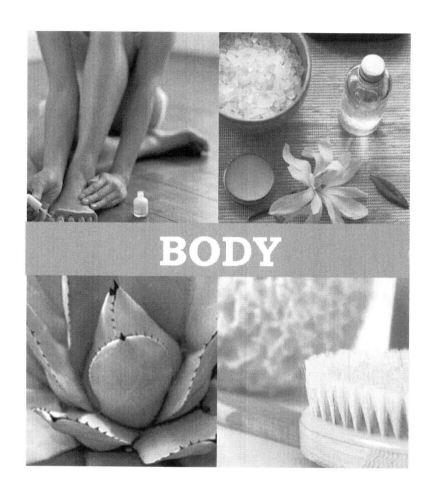

BODY

Beauty Tip: Natural mouthwash - Did you know that there's enough fluoride in green tea to reduce plaque and bacterial infections? Steep a green tea teabag in a cup of boiling water for 10 minutes. Then use as a mouthwash

61. Getting That Daily Glow

Looking radiant every day is easy if you know how. No amount of bronzer will give you the radiance that a natural glow can do. To achieve a natural glow it comes down to making a few lifestyle changes. Here is an example of how you can get a natural glow and become a natural beauty.

- Start the day off with a big glass of water and a few slices of lemon to kick start your system and help flush out any toxins.
- For breakfast feed your skin some antioxidants by having a bowl of fresh seasonal fruit topped with chia seeds and goji berries. If you are super hungry have one poached egg with a slice of whole meal toast.
- Go for a 30 minute walk, yoga or run to kick start your metabolism and get your blood circulating.
- When you get home make yourself a nourishing green smoothie. Blend some kale leaves, banana, coconut water and a pear together. Sip mindfully and feel the green power fuel your body.
- Before jumping in the shower do a little dry body brushing for an instant glow. Simply use a natural bristled body brush and work in gentle strokes towards your heart. This is great for removing toxins, reducing cellulite and buffing off dry skin.

- Now time for a shower and a little hot and cold therapy. Start the shower hot for 2 minutes than cold for 1 minute, do this a few times to get your circulation pumping. Doing this everyday will help firm and tone the skin and boost your immune system.

- While you are still in the shower give your body a scrub to get rid of any uneven dead skin cells and promote smooth glowing skin. You can use a natural scrub that you make yourself. Try mixing ½ cup sugar, 1/4 cup olive oil and 1 tsp. freshly grated ginger. Apply and rub into body. Please note: always patch test first.

- Moisturize your body with nourishing body oil and you are ready to start your day.

- Ensure that you drink two liters of water throughout the day to rehydrate and restore your body.

Beauty Tip: Refresh and Rehydrate – a great way to refresh your body is to sip on mint and lemon water. Simply add one tablespoon of fresh mint and two slices of lemon to a glass of water.

62. Summer Skin

So you want smooth, radiant skin for summer. Try these simple steps.

1. **Get lots of sleep**- your skin goes into rest and repair mode at night. That's when your skin works the most in repairing and healing.

2. **Freshen your face**- exfoliate your skin naturally with oatmeal scrub, add a little warm water to half a cup of oats to make a paste consistency, then massage over cleansed skin to remove dead skin cells.

3. **Hydrate**- drinking lots of water is essential for glowing summer skin. Aim to drink 2-3 liters.

4. **Green- juice each morning**. It gives your skin a big dose of vitamins, minerals, and amino acids.

5. **Use a fake tan**- it gives you that beautiful glow without those harmful rays...

6. **Eat for gorgeous skin**- Eat foods high in antioxidants such as berries, nuts and seeds. Also try eating foods that are rich in silica which include- green, leafy vegetables, cucumber, oats, whole grains and nettle tea.

7. **Dry body brush** - it encourages the flushing out of excess fluids and toxins. Evens skin tone works wonders for cellulite.

8. **Body scrub**- doing this a couple times a week will eliminate any dry and rough patches on your skin. It will also allow for

better absorption of body creams. Try making your own scrub.

63. Stretch marks

This is something that every woman, pregnant or not seeks a remedy for. Stretch marks are the result of a torn collagen bundles that occur when the skin is stressed. Here are some ways to heal and prevent stretch marks:

- Eat foods rich in vitamins C and E, zinc and essential fatty acids – they all assist in the production of collagen.
- Don't let your weight fluctuate too much. Steady weight gain and weight loss is always the best way.
- Consume at least one rich source of omega 3 per day, such as a piece of grilled salmon, a tablespoon of flaxseed oil, or a small handful of nuts and seeds.

64. Milk baths

Cleopatra bathed in milk because it contains proteins that soften the skin and lactic acid which helps dissolve superfluous skin cells. The milk also helps exfoliate the skin for additional softness. The milk bath provides relaxation for many people. The soothing feeling of milk in the water creates an overall relaxed, comfortable feeling. Relaxing in a milk bath at the end of the day can help you improve your skin whilst helping reduce the stress of your day.

To prepare a milk bath: Simply add two cups of milk to a bath - soak and enjoy.

Beauty Tip: Shower time bliss - next time after you have your shower or bath, treat yourself to a little face and body massage. Gently massage some olive oil or coconut oil into your skin. This will feed your skin whilst getting the blood flowing. It is a great remedy for treating cellulite and firming the skin. It will help relax you and prepare you for a blissful night's sleep.

65. Yoga for Beauty

Yoga cleanses the body, mind and soul. All the negative energy is cleared and you are left with more clarity. Yoga leaves you feeling blissed out and radiating with positivity. Yoga leaves you with a glow.

Yoga isn't just for relaxation, it can also turn back the clock. Yoga cultivates calm by driving down levels of stress hormones that cause havoc with your general health and skin. The beauty benefits of yoga are endless. Here is how:

- Through breathing techniques (pranayama) and physical postures (asana), yoga increases circulation which brings much needed nutrients and oxygen to your skin. This helps to rejuvenate and revitalize your skin.
- It switches on your internal calm, which then causes the facial muscles to relax. This reduces wrinkles and gives the face a natural lift.
- Through the postures; it encourages blood circulation. This allows more nutrients to be carried in the blood; therefore your body gets a nutritious boost.

- Several of the postures also provide a gentle massage to your internal organs, stimulating them to gradually release toxins. When you stimulate your lymphatic system your body can get rid of toxins more efficiently, which ultimately means clearer skin.
- Yoga postures can increase blood supply to the hair follicles in your scalp. The boost of nourishment creates thicker, shinier and healthier hair.

Beauty Tip: Want super soft hands! Massage some olive oil into your hands and nails. Then apply some cotton gloves and leave them on overnight.

66. Oil Pulling

Oil Pulling is an ancient Ayurvedic treatment that promotes self-healing within. It aids in removing toxins from your body, and once toxins are removed your body will glow with radiance. Oil pulling is simple, affordable and totally safe. It is a gentle 'do it yourself home remedy' that promotes health and wellbeing. Oil pulling simply involves rinsing your mouth with one tablespoon (10ml) of vegetable oil for 15 to 20 minutes and spitting it out.

67. Repair with Antioxidants

Give your diet an antioxidant boost with super purple berries such as Blueberries, Acai, or Camu Camu. Loaded with potent antioxidants, these super- berries protect cells from oxidative stress and premature ageing.

Try this berry buzz smoothie for a dose of antioxidants and protein

- 1 scoop of Acai berries
- 1 cup frozen organic berries
- 1 Banana
- 1 scoop natural protein powder
- 1 TBSP Ground Flaxseed
- 1TBSP Cinnamon
- 1 tsp. Spirulina Powder
- Water or coconut/almond milk to liquefy ingredients

68. Glow With Green Juice

Taking care of your skin is so important. Remember what you eat, drink and think about will show through your skin. You need to take care of yourself because you deserve it. One of the biggest beauty secrets is drinking a green smoothie or green juice every second day. It's so true - *the glow truly is in the greens*.

Green foods are among the most nutrient dense of all foods and are chock full of alkaline, minerals, chlorophyll and amino acids. Green foods are beauty foods as they regenerate, repair and purify your cells. By drinking a green juice every day you will drink your way to radiant skin, renewed energy and optimum health. Here is what green juices will do for you:

- Green drinks help you get a youthful radiant glow.
- Green drinks repair skin and diminish fine lines and wrinkles.
- Green drinks will help you grow lustrous hair and strong nails.
- Green drinks will flood your body with nourishment.

For a delicious and refreshing green juice try juicing together one pear, 2 cups of raw spinach, half a cucumber, half a lemon and a few sprigs of mint – it is divine.

Beauty Wisdom: *"The best and most beautiful things in the world cannot be seen or even touched - they must be felt with the heart."* - Helen Keller

69. Exfoliate To Radiance

You should aim to exfoliate once or twice a week. Your skin cells regenerate new skin cells every 30 days. Mature skin renews a lot slower, therefore exfoliation is strongly recommended for people with mature skin as the removal of

the surface dead cells encourages new cells to regenerate
Exfoliating the skin has so many wonderful benefits:

- Removes dead skin cells, grease and impurities from the surface of the skin.
- Removal of old skin improves the look of pigmentation, fine lines and flaws.
- Nutrients from moisturizers and body treatments are more easily absorbed into the skin.

Beauty Tip: Make your own mint and lime foot scrub

Ingredients:

- 3 limes
- 2 tbsp. sugar
- 1 tbsp. sweet almond oil
- 15 fresh Mint leaves (chopped)
- 5 drops lime essential oil

How to make - cut the limes into thin slices. Put all the lime pieces into a blender, blend to a pulp. Mix the lime pulp with almond oil, mint leaves and essential oil. Soak and reinvigorate tired feet.

70. Carrot Body Mask

Not only are carrots good for your health, they can tone and clarify your skin. Homemade masks made from carrots are soothing and nutritious for your skin. Carrots are a natural antiseptic which are bursting with vitamins (like carotene) and minerals. Carrots are affordable and readily available all year round at your local green grocer!

Make your own homemade carrot mask for your body (great for a face mask to):

- **Peel and steam carrots.** Peel five large carrots and steam or boil until tender (when a fork can easily pierce through it, it's ready). Mash the carrot with a fork until it's a creamy consistency.

- **Mix in a little honey and extra virgin olive oil.** Mix in 3 tablespoon of honey and 2 tablespoon of extra virgin olive oil. If your skin is oily, you may omit the extra virgin olive oil.

- **Add a few drops of lemon juice.** Your skin type will depend on the amount of lemon juice you add in (lemon juice is a natural astringent, so the oilier your skin, the more lemon you want in your mask). If you have dry skin, add about 15 drops of lemon and if you have oily skin, add up to 3 tablespoons.

- **Check the consistency.** The mixture shouldn't be too clumpy or too runny. If the mix is too thick, you can add in a bit more extra virgin olive oil or water to thin it out. You can add a bit more honey to the mix to give it a thicker, paste-like texture.

- **Mask time**. Apply the carrot mask onto your body, include your neck. Avoid the eye and mouth area if you are applying to face. Lie down on an old towel and turn on your favorite music and bliss out for 10 - 15 minutes while the mask nourishes your skin. Wash off with warm water. Pat dry and follow up with your favorite moisturizer.

Beauty Tip: Feeling tired? Yawn deeply and loudly. It's your body's natural way of getting oxygen to the body to increase vitality and clarity.

71. Soak In A Mud Bath

The healing properties of mud have been used for centuries too purify and detoxify the body. The high grade muds which are found in sea beds or in the earths ground are bursting with minerals that can easily be absorbed by your skin. Because of the purifying properties of mud – it promotes slimming and is often used in slimming body wraps. You can buy mud baths from good health food shops and beauty departments. Even though these baths seem uninviting they are extremely uplifting and nourishing. Sit in the bath for twenty minutes and let the goodness soak into your body, whilst you sip on a cleansing herbal tea to boost the detoxifying effects. Shower off quickly after woods, cozy up, rest and relax.

72. Essential Fatty Acids- Beautifying Fats

The reason these fats are called ' essential ' is that your body can't manufacture them; you must obtain them from foods you eat or through supplements. Essential Fatty Acids fall into two categories - Omega 3 and Omega 6.

So what are the skin beauty benefits of these fats?

- Stop fine lines from appearing and maintain hydrated and radiant skin.
- They have a powerful effect on our hormones, which makes us feel more balanced and does not stress the skin.
- Improve the blood flow in the body which means more nutrients are being released – resulting in a more nourished skin.
- They are a strong anti- inflammatory, which means they can fight skin infections and disorders such as acne and psoriasis.

- Your skin requires a constant supply of EFAs, but it particularly needs EFAs when stressed by the damage that occurs with sunburn.

Deficiency symptoms:

- Dry, scaly skin
- Eczema
- Inflammatory skin conditions
- Slow healing.
- Also hair loss or thinning, dandruff, splitting nails and dull hair.

73. Honey

Honey is a natural antibacterial and anti-inflammatory. It absorbs impurities from the pores and the skin. Ancient beauties used honey and milk on their skin regularly to keep their complexion looking young, radiant and smooth. You can use honey as a wash, toner or mask. And you can mix it with so many other ingredients depending on your needs. It's quite versatile.

Beauty Tip: Exfoliate your body to radiance – Use a handful of sea salt mixed with 1 tbsp. of wild lime juice and 3-4 drops of eucalyptus oil. Rub into the skin in a soft gentle circular motion from your feet to your chest and then up along your arms. Wrap yourself up in a warm towel or robe and await your bath.

74. The Sacred Healing Shower

Water has long been associated with healing and well-being, a relaxing bath, rejuvenating shower or an embracing ocean swim always leaves our bodies feeling reinvigorated and vibrant. Bask in the healing powers of water with the sacred shower. Put 3-4 drops of peppermint essential oil on a natural loofah or body clothe. Massage this into your skin with gentle circular movements. As you shower, bask in the falling water, let the water run off you and imagine that all your negative thoughts are being washed down the drain. Replace them with positive affirmations such as "I feel wonderful, nourished and alive"

Beauty Wisdom: Drink and eat with mindfulness – savor it *"Drink your tea slowly and reverently, as if it is the axis on which the world earth revolves – slowly, evenly, without rushing toward the future. Live the actual moment. Only this moment is life."* Thich Nhat Hanh

75. Dry Body Brush Yourself To Radiance

Grab a natural body brush or hemp mitt then lightly brush your skin starting at your feet. Move in a gentle sweeping movement towards your heart. Gradually make your way up your body and don't forget your arms, chest and neck. Body brushing stimulates the lymphatic system, helping to reduce fluid retention and removing toxins. As you body brush do not judge or criticize your body, brush it with love and nurture. Be grateful for how your body protects you and for what it allows you to do.

76. The Desert Journey Tea Bath

Soak in the aroma and tranquility of the Australian rainforest, this is a luxurious bath treat, guaranteed to leave you feeling calm and at one with nature.

You will need

- 1 tbsp. each of eucalyptus leaves, citrus peel, lavender, rosemary, chamomile and sage.
- 10 drops of lavender essential oil

To prepare put all the ingredients into a glass jar and shake, then add two tbsp. to a muslin bag or clothe, steep in the bath for a few minutes before getting in. You can keep the jar of the tea bath ingredients for up to three-six months. Now light some candles, put on some soothing music and let your mind get lost.

> **Beauty Tip**: Start the day with a few slices of lemon in a cup of hot water to kick start and stimulate your body for the day.

77. Detox Your Way To Beauty

If your energy levels are low, your hair and skin are dull and lacking luster and you have been over indulging lately - then maybe a detox is in order.

Detoxing is a part of any healthy lifestyle, by detoxing you are allowing your body to heal and repair itself. When you go on a detox your body is able to flush out all the toxins that build up throughout everyday modern living. Once your body is free from many toxins it then has the ability and energy to start repairing and healing other areas of your body such as illnesses, hair, skin, nails and everything else that may have been neglected.

To get started:

Start the day with a cleansing drink of lemon and water. Simply add the juice of half a lemon to a glass of warm water. This will aid in removing some toxins along with nourishing your body with Vitamin C and Potassium. Alternatively brew a cup of herbal tea if lemon is not your thing.

Cleansing foods:

- Avoid meat, dairy products, sugar, refined and processed foods, pasta, bread, rice, alcohol and coffee for the entire day.
- Increase your intake of fresh fruits, vegetables, juices and water.
- Drink at least two liters of water.
- Take 1000mg of antioxidant rich vitamin C to help cleanse and revitalize your system.
- Juice it - be sure to incorporate plenty of fresh vegetable and fruit juices, not only are they an excellent source of vitamins, minerals and fiber, they are also fabulous detoxifiers.

Detoxing Exercises

- Gentle yoga or Pilate's.
- A gentle walk in nature.
- A refreshing ocean swim.
- Detoxing DIY Spa Treatment

When it comes to feeling refreshed and reinvigorated a detox is a satisfying ritual. If the word detox sends shivers down your spine - then don't worry because you can still detox your body through a pampering body treatment. Try giving yourself an Epsom salt bath or a body wrap in mud.

78. Take an ocean swim

Take a moment to connect with nature and play in mother earth's best playground – the ocean. If you don't have an ocean near you then go to your local pool. Swimming is very therapeutic and it is a relaxing way to tone your body. This is your moment to connect with your mind, breath and inner wisdom. Spend 45 minutes connecting with the rhythm of your body, feel the minerals of the water nourishing your skin, bringing a radiant glow to your complexion.

Backstroke is very relaxing and is great for your shoulders.

Breaststroke is excellent for toning upper arms and inner thighs

Freestyle/front crawl is a great aerobic workout; this stroke tones the arms and works on the shoulders and upper back muscles.

79. A Seaweed Body Wrap

Take the time to indulge in the healing powers of the ocean – often referred to as Thalassotherapy. Inspired by the ocean, thalassotherapy uses water and marine extracts to heal and rejuvenate the body. Body wraps are one of the most popular treatments in spas due to their detoxifying properties. Seaweed has multiple benefits for the skin and body including firming, hydrating, and increasing the bodies circulation to aid in inner detoxification. A seaweed body wrap is also rich in negative ions which restores and re-energizes your body. Get ready to breathe in tranquility and bliss as you wrap yourself up in the warmth of a healing body wrap.

You will need

- 1 tsp. dried seaweed
- 250 ml of water
- 2 tbsp. kaolin clay
- 1 tbsp. rose water
- 2 tbsp. macadamia oil
- 1 tbsp. organic honey
- 1 drop of essential peppermint oil
- 2 drops of essential sandalwood oil
- 1 drop of essential lavender oil
- 1 drop of essential sage oil
- A Warm towel or sarong to wrap up in

Directions: Boil the seaweed in the water for five minutes and then leave to cool. Combine the kaolin, rose water, macadamia oil and the honey to the cooled water. Then add the essential oils. Mix together well.

Smooth the pack over your body and wrap yourself up in a warm towel or sarong. Leave on for twenty minutes. Rinse off under the shower

Beauty Tip: By drinking 2-3 liters of water, this will plump out fine lines and wrinkles and give your face a refreshed look.

80. Sweet Dreams

Sleep is one of the biggest contributors to beauty. Sleep is not a luxury it is a necessity to keep your body healthy, your energy bouncing and your beauty glowing. How many hours of sleep do you get at night? I hope your answer is between 7-8 hours per night.

Unfortunately many people underestimate the importance of sleep, if you are one of these, drop that thought now and schedule in more sleep time. Sleep should be a non-negotiable commitment in your holistic wellness plan if you want to be healthy, have energy, keep a stable weight, emit a radiant health glow and remain in a motivated and positive mind frame.

To get a good night's sleep it is a good idea to create a blissful wind down ritual. Use this one as a sample:

- Unwind with a cup of holistic delight – try a blend of cacao, stevia, coconut water, coconut milk and cashews and drink either cold or hot. Or if you prefer brew yourself a peppermint or chamomile tea.

- Light some candles put on some soothing music and soak in a lavender bath until your heart's content. When you have had enough, dry yourself off, rub in some more sweet almond oil and put on some clean pajamas.

- Before retiring for the day make sure you write down in your gratitude journal three things that you are grateful for.

- Put a CD on with ocean sounds, close your eyes, take a mindful breath and get lost in your dreams.

Beauty Wisdom: *"Sleep is the golden chain that ties health and our bodies together."* – Thomas Dekker

81. Apple Cider Vinegar

Apple Cider Vinegar not only has wonderful health benefits it is also a fantastic beautifier. Apple Cider Vinegar is super cheap and readily available. Not only is it great for you – it also won't harm the planet. Here are some ways you can start using Apple Cider Vinegar in your beauty routine today:

Beautiful Skin – Use it as a toner to help regulate and balance the PH level of your skin. Dilute one part of apple cider vinegar with two parts water and apply the soothing elixir to your face with a cotton wool ball. Great to use also in a bath.

Fade Blemishes and Scars - It is also wonderful at fading age spots, blemishes, stretch marks and acne scars. Simply apply a concentrated dab of apple cider vinegar on the blemish and leave overnight.

Whitening Teeth – Rub apple cider vinegar directly on your teeth to remove stains and brighten up your smile.

Detox Hair – Remove all the residue in your hair caused from the city smoke, traffic fumes and pollution. When used regularly in your natural hair care routine, apple cider vinegar will revitalize your hair, leaving it soft, shiny and smooth. Make up an apple cider vinegar hair rinse by mixing one part apple cider vinegar with one part water. After shampooing, pour the mixture onto your hair. If you have a spray bottle, that works even better. That way you can spritz your hair with the mixture and massage it into your scalp. Let the apple cider vinegar mixture sit for a few minutes before rinsing fully with water. No need to use conditioner.

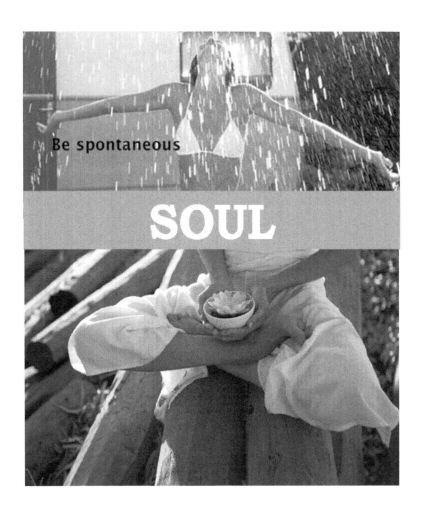

Be spontaneous

SOUL

Beauty Tip: It takes great courage to live your truth, but once you do your heart will open and you will be capable of great things.

82. Connect With Nature and Yourself

Dress in some comfy clothes and plan a leisurely walk in the park, by the beach, or at a nature reserve near your home. You are going to nurture yourself by taking a walk with a different point of view. Walk in awareness with soft eyes, feeling your connection to the Earth Mother. Look around and if something catches your eye like a bird, cloud or flower, take a moment to observe it more closely. See its simple beauty.

83. Spend The Evening In Self Love

Make your favorite herbal tea, burn your favorite essential oils and set your creative inspiration free. Create a vision board, a diary of possibilities or de-clutter a room to create space for new things to enter your life. Whatever you choose to do, do it fully with your heart - for when you live with purpose and passion, beauty will radiate from your entire being.

Beauty Wisdom: "And the day came when the risk it took to remain tight in the bud became more painful than the risk it took to blossom" – Anais Nin

84. Good vibrations

Listening to soothing sounds will instantly calm the mind and body. Harmonious tunes prompt the brain to release a hormone, known as ACTH (adrenocorticotropic hormone), which has a calming effect on the body. When you are calm and relaxed your beauty and wellness will be radiating. To relax effectively, listen to sounds of nature like the sea, rainforest, or birds singing. Classical music will also soothe and relax.

85. The Mystery Of Beauty

We all tend to focus far too much on how we look rather than how we feel. Our minds and souls need as much attention as our face and bodies! Both yoga and meditation create inner focus and calm. Some of the most attractive people have an internal brilliance – their eyes are bright and often sparkle, their skin has a subtle glow, they radiate an inner beauty which has nothing to do with their clothes, their weight or even their bone structure. It's an internal light that shines from within. For a woman to be beautiful, the inside must match the outside.

Beauty Tip: Stop making excuses. Have a bit of faith in yourself and drop all the reasons and excuses why it won't

100

work. Focus on how it can work. Yes it will be tough at times; however there are no shortcuts to success. If things are not working as you planned, re-evaluate, re-set goals, acknowledge your lessons and find a better way to do it.

86. Be Grateful

Live with a grateful heart and natural beauty will radiate from within you. When you choose to be grateful for what you do have, you shine with positivity, you attract abundance and you become much happier in life. Whatever it is that you don't like about yourself or your life – remember somebody else is doing it tougher somewhere else in the world. Take the time to write in a gratitude journal every night, write down three things that you are grateful for. Over time gratitude will become a natural habit in your everyday life.

Beauty Tip: It is time to regain your power, find your purpose and reignite that little flame within your own heart. The world needs you to be your best self – and you have waited long enough – YOU DESERVE TO BECOME YOUR BEST SELF AND LIVE YOUR BEST LIFE.

87. Don't Compare

Comparison is pointless; it wastes energy and does not bring out the best of you. When you compare yourself to other people, it is just your ego and self-doubt trying to convince you that you are not good enough, or are not doing things right. It is not your true reality; it is just your thoughts. You are on your own journey and you aren't supposed to replicate another person's life or look - you have your own unique role to fulfill in this world that no one else can. Release, surrender and trust the universe a little more. Ask for what you want, because you will be surprised at how often the universe says yes – you just have to ask first.

Beauty Tip: Create your own universe, live by your own rules and know that there is enough abundance and beauty for everyone in this world.

88. Listen To Your Inner Guidance

Take a moment to be alone and quiet the noise of the outside world. Drop all thoughts of expectations, release all the thoughts about caring what other people think and get deep into your heart, get silent and reconnect with your raw and authentic self. What does that voice within you say? What do you find beautiful? What do you believe is right and wrong? Get curious and ask your true self these questions, get to know your true self better. Once you start getting the answers, then start living your life this way. These answers are the key to knowing your passions and unlocking your true authentic self. The latest vogue magazine may say that blonde hair is beautiful but your inner self realizes that you find red hair beautiful. Find your truth and go live and express it. As Yves Saint Laurent once said *"The most beautiful make up of a woman is passion. But cosmetics are easier to buy"*

89. Remove the toxins

Take the time to try and remove as many toxins from your life as possible. This can be in the form of products, food, people, situations and thoughts. Remove the toxins and get in sync and balance with nature. Toxicity in your life weighs you down and makes you feel exhausted and dull. Replace toxic beauty products with natural ones. Replace sugary and high processed foods with more wholefoods. Stop spending time with people that drain your energy and make you feel like crap. Replace all your negative and self-limiting beliefs with more positive statements.

Beauty Tip: You are unique and needed. The world needs you to own your strengths so that you can serve and inspire others.

90. Embrace And Accept Yourself

You were created unique and it is your differences that make you beautiful. Choose to embrace and love who you are – flaws and all. It is far more beautiful to see a woman embrace her authentic self as opposed to trying to be a bad carbon copy of the girl in the magazine.

Learn to love who you are, see the beauty in your flaws, for they are raw, earthy and natural. You were created as part of nature, and everything in nature is beautiful and perfect. If you find yourself thinking that you do not like something about your natural self, ask yourself "what is it that I do like?" For example you may think your natural brown hair color is dull and boring. Switch your focus and appreciate how soft and healthy it is because it is not dry and brittle from over-coloring.

Choose to see the beauty behind what you find average or dull. Choose to see the extra-ordinary in the everyday ordinary. You will be surprised how much beauty surrounds you every day – you just need to look. Everything is perfect just as it is – for that is how nature intended it to be.

91. Dare To Be Different

Don't be like everybody else; break free of all those ideologies, theories and labels, for they don't serve you well. The world needs to hear your truth, be brave and go speak and live your truth. Daring to live with passion and authenticity is not for the faint hearted - for many people will not understand you. However by living your truth you set yourself free and you make the world a better place.

Beauty Tip: Have your own rules. Define what success looks like for you then go after it. We were all created different for a reason. Find your reason and use it.

92. Find Your Passion

To be beautiful is to be happy, people that are happy inspire the world, and they make the world a beautiful place. So how do you find your happy?

The heart of true happiness only begins to beat when you discover something that moves you, frees you, challenges you and gives you a sense of purpose. True happiness lies in taking the time to discover your passion and then pursuing it with an open heart. Discovering your passion is a lifelong journey, one with many twists and turns, it is about slowly rediscovering who you truly are. Go searching for that one thing that makes you come alive. Become it, breathe it and let it become you. When you live like this, great things will happen for you, to you and because of you. And if you don't know what your passion is – get curious and follow anything that intrigues you, for it may just take you somewhere new.

Take the time to discover and ignite your passion (or follow your curiosity) and get your heart beating back to the rhythm of happiness – for this is the moment that beauty becomes you.

Beauty Tip: Change your focus. The secret to doing things to uplift you is to know your strengths. Instead of focusing on what you are not good at, focus on what you are good at.

93. Work For A Purpose

In June 2005, Steve Jobs took to the stage at Stanford Stadium to give a speech to Stanford's graduating class. He addressed a crowd of 23 000, drawing on lessons that he learnt. About halfway through the speech Jobs offered the following wisdom:

"Your work is going to fill a large part of your life, and the only way to be truly satisfied is to do what you believe is great work. And the only way to do great work is to love what you do. If you haven't found it yet, keep looking. Don't settle. As with all matters of the heart, you'll know when you find it. And, like any great relationship, it just gets better and better as the years roll on. So keep looking until you find it. Don't settle." - Steve Jobs

This famous quote from Steve Jobs stirs something deep within most of us. It sparks the idea of happiness, fulfillment, meaning and purpose. We all want to feel happy and enjoy what we are doing. However many of us are tired and exhausted, we no longer know where to look for our true happiness. We seek high and low, only to come full circle and end up where we left off.

You need to go out into the world and search for a job that sparks your soul and makes you feel alive. For when passion and skill come together, the end result is often a masterpiece. Pursue a career that is meaningful to you, not because the paycheck is big. Most of us have to work for a living, why not turn hard work into play. If you cannot find a job that you love – then create one. Yes this can be scary stuff; however success only comes to those who actually try and not to those who just sit and wonder.

If by chance you have set out to start up your own business, but feel like giving up – whatever you do, do not give up. The world is a huge place and it is only a matter of time before you find someone who will love and appreciate your work.

94. Never Give Up

No matter how bad things get, never let yourself get discouraged. Often when we set out to pursue our dreams the road leads us on another path. Never give up, trust that you will be shown the right path that is meant for you. Have faith is the madness, and know that the universe has grander plans for you. Often where you plan to go is not where you end up. Trust the process.

95. Make A Difference

When you are committed to following your dreams and trying something new, you radiate with positivity and love. People feel your passion, are moved by your passion and are inspired by your passion. Through your strength and authenticity you will inspire other people to go take daring leaps and follow their own dreams.

96. Drop the Fear

There is no beauty to be found in settling for a life that you are not passionate about. You only get one chance, so make today count. Stop consuming yourself with what others will think, loosen the grip on all those preconceived ideas, for at the end of the day nothing matters more than your own happiness.

97. Say "Yes" To Life

There is no such thing as luck - people that seem to have it all have generally worked very hard. You must endlessly seek and build opportunities. No matter who you are, nobody stumbles across the perfect life or dream job – it takes time and perseverance to build the perfect life or dream job. Remember that nothing is ever as it seems, there is a whole lot more going on than you could ever know behind what seems "ever so perfect". Find new opportunities by opening your heart and saying "yes" to life.

98. Fill Your Life With Beauty

You have more room in your life to move than you have ever imagined. You need to clear the clutter, and then rebuild it with things that energize you. Consciously choose things that inspire you and drop the things that don't. If there is a non-negotiable in your life that drains you, one that you cannot drop – then choose to look at it from a different perspective. Choose to see the good in it, the lessons learnt and the beauty in it – after all everything in life has some beauty – sometimes we just choose not to see it.

Follow the 25 per cent rule. Fill your life with mostly things that invigorate you. Dedicate 25% per cent of your day to things that you don't enjoy (difficult conversations, dealing with grumpy customers, etc.) and dedicate the rest of the day focusing on doing things that uplift you.

Beauty Tip: Get back to simplicity - all too often we live our lives in reverse. We work hard to acquire more stuff, to make more money, to get that promotion. We often think that by getting all this stuff we will be able to do more of what we want, we think this stuff will bring us happiness. Often we are living life backwards, when all we really need to do is live more mindfully by simply doing more things that we love.

99. Live For The Moment

Be open, aware and present. Live today as if it is your last and look for all the miracles that surround you. If you open your ears, eyes and heart the world will teach you more and more about who you really are. The secret to finding your best self is to look within the here and now – sometimes you just have to change your perspective and know where to look.

100. Focus On Your Strengths

To spark your inner beauty is to understand your strengths and know what inspires you. Trust yourself and don't let other people tell you what you are good and bad at. Don't look to your parents, teaches or bosses to tell you who you are. Your strengths and weaknesses are not defined in your bosses employee review, customer feedback form or in what people say about you.

Sometimes you may be good at something, but you don't enjoy it. Only you know your true strengths and weaknesses. A weakness is any activity that makes you feel weaker and depleted. Your strengths make you feel in focus. When you are tapped into your strengths you feel like time goes by super-fast, you feel focused, energized and in the zone. Your greatest clue to finding your strengths is to ask yourself "Do I feel energized before, during and after the activity". Anything that leaves you feeling otherwise, you need to find ways to drop it and replace it.

Your greatest opportunities for growth come out of your strengths and not your weakness. You are more challenged, focused and successful when you focus more on what you are good at and what you enjoy.

So what do you do with your weakness? You never try and fix your weaknesses; instead you find a way to make them irrelevant by making your strengths more productive. If you focus on your strengths you naturally over time grow and improve on your weaknesses. Follow your strengths and your path will naturally heal your weaknesses.

As you grow you intensify who you really are. You get wiser, more resilient, a clearer perspective and more worldly – but you never change the core of who you really are – weaknesses and strengths. You have always had the power and everything you need within you. The real challenge is to make you the most productive version of who you really are by focusing on your strengths.

Beauty Tip: Add more spark into your life by getting intentional and doing one thing every week for the rest of your life that uplifts you. Find something that makes you feel good and spend the week focusing on it and find ways to implement it into your day. This will make you sharper and more vibrant, it will help pull you out of the wrong space and put you in the right space. Do this for the rest of your life.

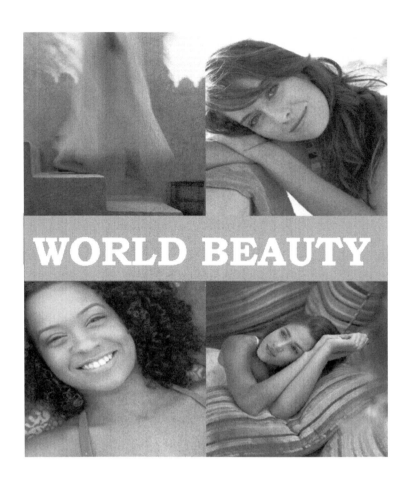

WORLD BEAUTY

Indian Beauty Secrets

Within the ancient lands of India there lie many ancient beauty secrets that the women of India have been using for years. The secrets are both ancient and proven. Indian women have relied on the powers of nature and herbs for over 2000 years. Mothers have passed on their beauty secrets to their daughters to help make them become an Indian princess.

Indian women mostly focus on their complexions, body shape and hair care. They love to nurture their hair, look after their skin and build curves on their body. Here are some sacred secrets to becoming an Indian princess.

Greet the sun. Wake up before sunrise, it is a great way to balance and harmonize your body. Try doing a few sets of the Sun Salutation yoga poses to get your body warmed up, circulation pumping and energy flowing.

Discover herbs. Include herbs like turmeric and ginger in your daily diet, as these have antiseptic properties that will not only help fight illness but also help with any skin inflammation and premature ageing.

Spice it up. If you are on a journey to lose weight, you may want to spice it up by adding a little chili to your meal. Chilies speed up your metabolism and help flush out toxins.

Go crazy for bananas. If you would like help fighting fine lines and wrinkles then mash up a banana and apply it as a facemask. Leave on for 15 minutes.

Chickpea magic. To tone and even out your skin wrap your body in a chickpea body wrap. Make a paste of chick pea flour, turmeric and milk. Add the ingredients until it has a thick consistency. Apply this paste all over your body and gently massage it in with a circular motion. Wrap yourself in an old blanket and bliss out for 15 minutes. Wash it off after 10-15 minutes.

Refresh with cold water. Every morning and evening after washing your face, splash your face with cold water. This helps to close the pores whilst improving your blood circulation and cell renewal.

Treat acne prone skin. An old ritual that has been used by Indian women for years to treat acne is the sandalwood and turmeric face mask. Mix a few drops of sandalwood oil with 1 teaspoon of turmeric powder. Then mix the paste into 1 cup of natural yoghurt. Apply the mask to your face and wash it off after 15 minutes. This mask has anti-septic properties, which will help make your skin smooth, soft and acne-free.

Mystery eyes. Ancient Indian women used Kajal (homemade natural eyeliner) to define their eyes. It is made from castor oil, coconut oil, almond oil and black mustard seeds. This formula helps to make your eyes brighter and whiter, whilst improving your vision and stimulating the growth of eye lashes.

Hair like silk. Indian women take a lot of pride in maintaining their sleek hair. They prefer to use natural ingredients such as coconut oil and henna. For a nourishing hair mask simply massage either coconut oil or henna into your hair for 15 minutes and then wash out. It will repair your hair along with encouraging it to grow faster.

The ancient practices of Ayurveda. Ayurveda is an Indian form of medicine where they focus on healing the body by connecting with nature. Ayurveda advises to not put anything on your skin that you cannot eat. Indian women like to make their own beauty treatments as they believe it helps harmonize the body with nature.

Be happy. Indian women know that being beautiful will not make them happy, so instead they focus on being beautiful from the inside out. They believe in being grateful for everything they have and appreciating the small things in life. In the land of India, a smile is one of the greatest beauty secrets.

A mother's secret. This ancient beauty treatment has been passed down from mother to daughter for years. The honey and cinnamon mask is a traditional ritual that has proven to work. Simply mix together 1-2 tablespoons of honey with 1 teaspoon of cinnamon. Apply as a face mask and wash off after 15 minutes.

Korean Beauty Secrets

When it comes to skincare products South Korea is the new France. Their products are innovative and highly advanced, making South Korea one of the most advanced and leading beauty capitals in the world. Korean women are known for their flawless skin; in fact you could go as far as saying that obtaining perfect skin is almost an obsession for many Korean women.

"Bright skin meant that you came from a noble family" says Dr. Seung Yoon Celine Lee, a dermatologist based in Seoul.

Korean women have perfectly toned, plump and youthful skin. So what is their secret? Firstly they eat a lot of fresh fish and vegetables and secondly they spend hours and money priming and prepping their skin to perfection.

One of the things that Korean women do is that they perform an intense facial routine every morning and night. This process is not for the faint hearted or penny-pincher. It takes a lot of time and products to achieve the Korean perfection. So if you have a spare five minutes, let me demystify their beauty routine and go through with you step-by-step and product-by-product.

1. **Start with double cleansing the face**. Korean women believe that washing your face once is not enough.

The first cleanse is to remove any makeup and residue. Start with wiping your face over with some cleansing wipes or by using a makeup removing facial wash. The second wash is to deep cleanse and purify the pores. Use a professional cleanser formulated for your skin type.

2. **Next tone the face**. Use a toner with cold water to wipe off any residue, prep the skin and close up the pores.

3. **Time for a little essence**. I can hear you say what on earth is essence? Essence is a fancy word used for a rose facial spritzer. The purpose of essence is to hydrate the skin and prep it for moisturizing and nourishing.

4. **Emulsion**. Emulsion is a product you use before you apply your moisturizer. The emulsion helps to absorb the nutrients once the moisturizer is applied.

5. **Serum**. Serum is a concentrated hydrating/regenerative skin treatment. Serum is the super food for the skin, jam packed with all the vitamins and minerals needed for skin repair.

6. **Moisturizer.** Ahh about time…. after all that we are finally here. Moisturizer seals the skin and locks in the moisture and vitamins. This is also the time where Korean women apply a whitening cream and sunscreen.

7. **Eye Cream**. Time for a little eye pampering. Since your eyes are usually the first things to show signs of fatigue and age, it is vital that you take proper care of this thin part of your skin. Invest in an eye cream and don't use your regular moisturizer. Using your regular face moisturizer is too heavy for the eye area and will clog the delicate part around your eyes causing little white pimples under the eye. Eye creams are specially formulated to be lighter and more suited to this delicate area.

8. **Weekly maintainers**. Korean women swear by face masks once a week and facial massages every night to keep their skin glowing. Korean women also indulge in regular visits to the spa; in fact it is rare to find a Korean woman who has never been to a spa, as it's a huge part of their culture and health.

In the process of this exhaustive skin care routine Korean women strive for white and pure skin. To help them get this porcelain look they use a combination of whitening products, laser, photo facials along with various products to help remove blemishes.

Sun protection is also a big part of the Korean beauty regime and you will often find the Korean beauties walking outdoors with umbrellas, hats and wearing sunscreen is a non-negotiable must.

"Koreans aren't about stripping the skin until it looks like something you want to ice skate on. They're into nurturing it," says Schook, who also introduced eyelash extensions to New York almost a decade ago.

Korean women use on average 16-18 products a day, some of the popular products that these women love to nourish their skin with are:

The skin plumping mask and serum. This is an advanced formula that repairs bone and tissue on a surface level. It is like botox in a cream. The medical grade formula is in high demand worldwide and is slowly being introduced to clinics across the globe.

BB Cream. The Blemish Balm Cream is amongst Korea's hottest beauty products. The original formula was designed in Germany where dermatologists used it for healing scars caused by laser skin surgery. The soothing and regenerative properties of this miraculous cream have Korean women using it daily. It also doubles as a tinted moisturizer.

Whitening creams. In Asian countries a blemish free complexion along with a fair skin tone is considered beautiful. Korean women use a whitening cream 1-2 times daily to remove skin yellowness, freckles blemishes or scars. Korean women believe a perfect complexion involves having fair skin and consider it more important in their beauty routine than wearing makeup.

Japanese Beauty Secrets

If Italian women make the best lovers and French women are elegant, then Japanese women should be labeled as ageless. It might be the copious amounts of fresh fish, or the fact they use umbrellas to hide away from the sun's rays. Or maybe their timeless beauty is achieved through their kooky beauty secrets. Find out how you too can get that youthful glow with these not so mainstream beauty treatments. Here is what Japanese women swear by:

Seaweed. To get their translucent glow Japanese women use cleansers and toners that are made with seaweed essence. Seaweed gives the skin a glow whilst reducing the pore size. They don't just stop at their skin care; they also bath in it, wrap in it and eat it. Make your own seaweed bath by adding 1 cup of dried seaweed to a warm bath. Seaweed is great for drawing out the toxins.

Oranges. If you crave the fresh and sunny complexion that Japanese women have, then you need to increase your uptake on oranges. Oranges help reduce the melanin pigment from your skin to give you a bright and refreshed face. Either drink fresh orange juice every couple of days or apply the pulp and juice of one orange to your face like a mask. Leave on for 15 minutes.

Adzuki. There is a sacred Japanese ritual that has been used by Japanese women for years. They crush adzuki beans and rub it on their face. This helps to keep the skin free from blemishes and also improves the smoothness and tone of their complexion.

Rice Bran Wash. Rice bran is used as a wonderful way to refresh and rejuvenate your skin and prevent the signs of premature aging. A rice bran wash or otherwise known as Komenuka works at fading wrinkles and dark circles.

Wakame Kelp. This sea algae has healing properties which protect your skin from dirt, sun and pollution. It is also great at guarding against fine lines and wrinkles and fading dark circles.

Nightingale Droppings. This one is a little kooky. Japanese women pay to have facials that use the feces of nightingales. This facial is known as Uguisu, and it's naturally occurring enzyme leaves skin soft and supple.

Goldfish. To remove the dead skin cells from feet, Japanese dip their feet into a small pond of tiny toothless fish. This is a common practice where hundreds of tiny fish nibble at your feet for about 15 minutes, eating away all the dirt and dry skin, giving you clean and soft feet.

Bull Semen. Yes you did read it right. The semen of the bull is rich in protein and used as a conditioning mask for hair. That definitely is a different way to repair your dry ends.

Silkworm Cocoons. A common Japanese practice is to visit a spa and have a silkworm body scrub. They use the worm's cocoons to buff and polish their skin to perfection.

Daily Walk. Japanese are health conscious people, they believe in healthy walks on a daily basis to help tighten up the skin and oxygenate the body.

Sip on Green Tea. Japanese people drink several cups of green tea every day. Green tea is rich in antioxidants which help slow down the aging process and keep the skin youthful and supple.

Healthy Diet. Japanese are well known for their healthy cuisine. Their staple diet includes fish, which is very high in Omega-3, which helps promote healthy and glowing skin.

Brazilian Beauty Secrets

Brazilian women are among the most beautiful women in the world and have long been recognized as natural goddesses.

What to look a little like Giselle? Then try these tips to become a Brazilian Goddess.

Babassu Oil. Babassu oil is native to Brazil and is derived from the Babassu tree. Babassu oil is similar to coconut oil. Babassu oil is semi-solid at room temperature, and melts like silk when applied to the warmth of your skin. When applied it creates a beautiful cooling feeling on your skin, leaving it deeply nourished and moisturized.

Acai Berries. Brazilian beauties can thank the acai berry for their beautiful Brazilian glow, for the have been eating these berries for years. They either eat them as they are or put them in their morning fruit smoothie. These little berries are ranked as one of the best super foods; research has proven that they are one of the most nutrient rich foods available in the world. Acai (ah-sigh-ee) is the high-energy berry of a special Amazon palm tree. Harvested in the rainforests of Brazil, acai tastes like a vibrant blend of berries and chocolate. Acai is a jam packed full of antioxidants, amino acids and essential fatty acids. Although acai may not be available in your local supermarket, you can find it in your local health food shop.

Sand. If you are lucky enough to live near a warm sandy beach, try rubbing a little sand on your body. It acts as a natural exfoliant, buffing your skin to Brazilian perfection, leaving it ultra-soft and smooth. Wash the sand off in the healing salt water.

Brazilian Wax. The Brazilian bikini wax is perhaps the most well-known Brazilian beauty tip. Brazilian women prefer a cleanly waxed bikini area so that they can wear their latest bikini with style. Salons around the globe routinely perform this service.

Sugaring. Sugaring is a way that Brazilian women remove unwanted hair. The sugaring mixture can be used for Brazilian bikini waxing, upper lip waxing, eyebrow waxing, forearm waxing, underarm waxing, leg waxing, etc.

You can do it at home with this simple homemade recipe. You will need 2 cups sugar, 1/4 cup lemon juice (freshly squeezed) and 1/4 cup water. Simply boil down the mixture until it becomes a thick paste. Allow the mixture to cool enough to apply to the unwanted hair.

Use the mixture as you would with any hair removal wax. Cut old bed sheets into strips and press them down over the sugar solution on your skin. Hold surrounding skin taught and PULL!

Be confident. Not all Brazilian women look like Gisele; however they all seem to ooze sex appeal. Brazilian women love who they are and they own their beauty. Brazilian beauty is all about a positive attitude.

Brazilian keratin. A word that often leaves the lips of Brazilian women is "escova progressiva" – known as the "progressive blow dry." This blow wave is what is referred to the rest of the world as the Brazilian Keratin - a hair straightening treatment. The treatment turns frizzy hair into silky and smooth locks for up to six months. The process involved in this treatment is known as progressive blow dry treatment. The hair is sealed with keratin and heat to make the hair glossy and straight. The original Brazilian keratin treatment has been banned in many countries due to the formula containing Formaldehyde, a product that is proven to cause cancer. However today there is available many natural and 100% Formaldehyde-free treatments. Whilst these more natural treatments only last 3-4 months they are not only cheaper but they are much safer for you. Opt for the safe and natural treatment to get beautiful shiny hair like the Brazilian women.

Acai fruit oil. Acai fruit oil is another add-on to the list of Brazilian beauty tips. Acai fruit oil can either be purchased as an oil or it can be made at home by simply making a paste of acai fruit and applying it on your skin. Many Brazilian beauties apply this paste daily and wash it off after 30 minutes. This paste gently removes any dead skin cells, polishing the skin to a beautiful healthy glow.

African Beauty Secrets

The vast and rugged plains of Africa are one of the world's most extreme places. Days are often hot, dry and harsh. For centuries African women have had to find ways to fight the dehydrating effects of their harsh and unpredictable land. So from mother to daughter beauty secrets were passed down. Here are a few ancient beauty secrets from the land of Africa.

Black Soap. Black Soap, also known as Ose DuDu, is an organic soap from West Africa. The ingredients consist of essential oils, shea butter, plantain skins, palm oil, and coconut oil. Black soap has long been used to heal problem skin. It's great for reducing fine lines, evening out dark spots, eczema, razor bumps and eliminating blemishes. It is also used to lightly exfoliate and give you healthier looking skin. The natural exfoliating properties leave the skin fresh, supple and renewed. Black soap can be found online or in local beauty stores and is extremely affordable.

Shea Butter. Shea butter's success has crossed the frontiers of Africa where it was once originally used by African women to nourish their skin and hair. Shea butter, also known as karite, comes from the nut of the Karite Tree in Africa. Shea butter restores and moisturizes the skin, leaving the skin soft, velvety and supple.

Kaolin Clay. Kaolin is another star ingredient from Africa that has been used as a beautifier for years. Women have been using kaolin for centuries to nourish dry skin and pull out any impurities. African women also applied the white clay as a hair mask to help revitalize their sun damaged hair.

Rooibos. Rooibos is an amazing natural active ingredient to help fight irritated and inflamed skin such as acne, rosacea or eczema. Rooibos is brimming with powerful antioxidants, zinc, copper, rutin and alpha hydroxy acids. This makes rooibos ideal for treating all fungal infections, sensitive skin and premature ageing. Women in South Africa would steep a cup of rooibos in hot water, allow it to cool, and then topically apply the liquid to the skin with a cotton ball. The tannins in the tea would soothe and relieve discomfort. Rooibos can be drunk as a tea – it truly is a great beautifier from the inside out.

Baobab. This odd looking tree is often referred to as the "tree of life", because it provides everything from water, food and shelter. The baobab tree produces a fruit which is fast on its way to being dubbed the next "super fruit". The fruit contains 10 times higher antioxidant levels and 6 times more vitamin C than oranges. It also contains calcium, zinc, magnesium and most importantly omegas 3, 6 and 9. This makes it a priceless natural ingredient in anti-aging skincare regimens. When used in skincare the baobab fruit helps boost collagen production resulting in a smooth and youthful glow.

Honey. Women in South Africa lathered their bodies and hair in a mask of honey to nourish and beautify. Honey is a wonderful natural beauty product as it hydrates the skin and hair by sealing in moisture and locking in the nutrients. Honey is also a natural antioxidant and anti-microbial ingredient, so it helps protect the skin from the sun's damaging rays and supports cell rejuvenation and replenishment.

Try this South African Hair Mask Recipe to nourish and repair your hair.

You will need

- A little olive oil
- 1 egg yolk
- Honey

Coat your hair with the mask. Place a shower cap over your hair and relax for around 30 minutes. The heat from your head will help to make the nutrients from the hair mask really sink into your hair. Wash out thoroughly and you will be left with beautiful soft and shiny hair.

Australian Beauty Secrets

Australian women are legendary sand-and-sea beauties. With a culture that is so focused on sand, sun and fun – I hit up these bronzed beauties from down under, to find out what is on their must have beauty list.

Tea Tree Oil. Australian women apply tea tree oil to their hair, which helps nourish it and prevents dandruff. The best way to do this is to simply add a few drops of tea tree oil to your shampoo. Mixing tea tree oil in a moisturizer and applying on acne prone skin works wonders for relieving and healing the inflammation.

Paw Paw Ointment. One of Aussie women's best kept secrets is a tube of paw paw ointment. Paw Paw ointment is a natural remedy used to treat a multitude of ailments including everything from burns and cuts, to dry skin and chapped lips. Almost every Aussie woman has a tube of this ointment in her handbag, as it is great for nourishing the lips. Paw paw can be used topically to treat pimples, sunburn, boils, bruises, chafing, cuts, burns, cysts, dry patches, cracked skin, chapped lips, insect stings, mosquito bites and splinters, among many other ailments.

Zinc Cream. Australia is hot and has the highest rate of skin cancer, so people in Australia have to be extra vigilant about sun protection. Zinc is the ultimate skin shield; it goes on like a thick white mask, creating a barrier from the sun.

Sunshine. The Australian lifestyle revolves around the beach and the great outdoors, and the reason that Aussies look so healthy is that they get a good dose of sunlight every day. Sunlight infuses the body with vitamins and energy, causing you to feel revitalized, healthy and inspired

Laughter. Australia is known as being carefree and relaxed. The Aussie laid back lifestyle tends to be less stressful and more focused on fun. The culture of Australia is to have a good laugh and enjoy yourself – after all life is to short not to. One of the greatest beauty secrets to come from this country is to radiate happiness through laughter and living with a zest for life. Laughter is the greatest antidote for beauty.

Reduce cellulite. With the culture of sun, sand and fun many Australian women spend more time in swimwear than in their normal everyday clothes. With their bronzed and tanned bodies they look flawless in their bikinis, no lumps, bumps and cellulite. So how do these Australian beauties do it? Here is what they do to banish cellulite:

1) Avoid processed foods and refined sugar, and eat a diet high in brown bread, brown rice, pasta, potatoes, vegetables, diary, lean meat and fruit.

2) Consume lean protein sources like egg whites, poultry, fish and lean red meats.

3) Hydrate their bodies and skin with 2-3 liters of water a day, which prevents fluid retention in fat and makes their skin glow.

4) Dry body brush from head to toe every day before their morning shower. This gets the circulation flowing and helps remove toxins and therefore helps reduce cellulite.

5) Eat a diet rich in good fats such as olive oil, nuts and avocadoes.

6) Eat plenty of fiber rich foods. Whole foods are good sources of fiber and help lower the absorption of fats, and contribute to the regulation of the intestine.

7) Get 8 hours of sleep every night. Sleep balances out the hormones and helps the body fight fat.

8) Take time out from the stress of life. Many Australians do yoga and meditation to help them de-stress. When the body is in stress mode it naturally holds on to fat as a backup source. The less you stress the easier it is to fight fat.

9) Take a multi-vitamin and vitamin C supplement. When the body does not get all the nutrients that it needs, which is easier in today's world full of depleted soils, the body goes

into starvation mode and holds on to fat. Ensure that you are getting all the nutrients that you need by giving your body a boost with a high-grade supplement.

10) Get the heart pumping by doing some type of aerobic exercise to promote fat burning, such as hiking, biking, and swimming.

Italian Beauty Secrets

Italian women exude mystery, confidence and class, they have looking good down to a fine art. Here are a few luxury secrets that Italian women have used for years to seduce the world.

Fresh Food. Italian women eat a diet rich in fresh and healthy ingredients like olive oil, fresh fish, whole grains and vegetables. They consume fresh produce and enjoy red wine that is filled with antioxidants. Their healthy, balanced diet not only helps maintain a trim waistline, it also gives them gorgeous glowing skin, shiny hair and healthy nails.

Walking. These Italian beauties walk everywhere; the culture in Italy is to walk wherever you need to go. Daily trips to the market ensure that they are getting their heart pumping and circulation flowing. People who walk at least thirty minutes a day will not just look better, but they will feel much happier.

Healthy Hair. How do Italian women maintain their glossy locks? The answer is right in your kitchen. Italian women keep their hair shiny by feeding their hair with a mask of yogurt and olive oil - using the mixture as a deep conditioning treatment. To make this nourishing treatment at home, simply mix 1 cup of plain whole-milk yogurt with 1 teaspoon olive oil. Then apply the mixture to washed hair, let it sit for 5 minutes and rinse with cool water.

Olive Oil. Italians use olive oil for everything - olive oil is rich in healthy fats that help repair the body. For optimum health and a glowing complexion use olive oil on top of your salads, chargrilled vegetables and cured meats, and for an extra kick get in the routine of swallowing one tablespoon daily.

Italian women also used olive oil as part of their daily beauty routine. To repair damaged hair apply 1/3 cup of olive oil to the entire length of your hair, wrap a warmed towel around your hair and leave to rest for 20 minutes. Rinse well. This is a great remedy for fizzy hair and split ends.

For cracked feet rub the olive oil onto your feet before going to sleep and put on a pair of cotton socks. In the morning you will have soft and healthy feet.

Rosemary. Another important beauty remedy is rosemary – Italian women would use it as a clarifying face mask for oily skin. To make this herbal elixir, take a few fresh rosemary sprigs and boil them for five minutes with a cup of water. Strain the rosemary water to remove the leaves and then add the juice from one lemon. Whisk it all together. Apply on your face, leave for 15 minutes and wash away.

Coffee. Italy is famous for its coffee; the freshly brewed aroma is a delight for the senses. Italian women not only gracefully sip on their cups of coffee at artesian cafes they also use it as a scrub to remove cellulite. The coffee helps stimulate circulation to help remove toxins and the scrubbing helps to tighten and smooth the skin. Make the coffee sugar honey scrub by combining ½ cup coffee grinds with ¼ cup of brown sugar and 3 tablespoons of honey. Place olive oil over areas of cellulite and rub the mix for 5 minutes to exfoliate. Repeat 2-3 times a week and over time you will see your cellulite improve.

Tomatoes. A roma facial is one of the best beauty secrets of Italian women. Since tomatoes are in abundance in Italy, Italian beauties take advantage of this natural beauty product. A roma facial will hydrate and feed your skin, leaving you with an enviable glow. The best part is that a roma facial is super easy to do and very affordable. To give yourself this Italian treatment, simply slice a tomato into thin strips. Apply a thin layer of yogurt or milk all over your face avoiding the eye and mouth area. Carefully sit the sliced tomato on your face where you have applied the yogurt. A bonus tip is to apply some cool cucumber slices on your eyes to soothe puffiness and reduce dark circles. Take a moment to unwind by burning some beautiful oils and listening to some soothing music, allow the Roma facial to feed your skin for about 10 to 15 minutes then wash it off with lukewarm water.

Tomatoes are bursting with goodness and they are great for soothing any skin inflammation or irritation. Yoghurt provides intense hydration to the skin.

Moroccan Beauty Secrets

Moroccan women are known for using the gift of nature to beautify and care for every bit of their body. This beauty regime deprived from nature brings them a deep sense of well-being and an undisputed natural glow.

The secrets of how to get the best from botanicals and herbs is an art that is whispered from mother to daughter, down through the generations. Together let's take the journey through the world of well-being and beauty, while also discovering the heart and soul of Morocco.

Enchanted Bathing Rituals. The women of Morocco regularly escape the stress of the day by retreating into a blissful bath. They wash and exfoliate themselves to perfection in the warmth of the candlelight. Many like to add rose petals or essential oils such as rose, orange flower or sandalwood. Temporally they leave the world behind as they get lost and enchanted by the sensuality of the music that plays in the background and soothes their soul.

Henna. Henna is an old Moroccan beauty secret that has stood the test of time. Henna is commonly known to be used for temporary tattoos; however Moroccan beauties also use it on their hair and body as a nourishing beauty treatment. A common treatment is to use henna as a body wrap to diminish pimples, blackheads and all impurities whilst giving an instant glow to the skin. Try this Moroccan body wrap:

1. First exfoliate your body with a natural mit or body brush.
2. Purchase the white henna which you can find at any Middle Eastern store and most health shops. Ask for the light colored henna that doesn't dye your skin.
3. Mix the henna with fresh lemon juice and then add some water to make it into a thin consistency.
4. Apply to your entire body and wait about 10 minutes. Don't worry if you get a slight tingling sensation, as it is just the henna and the lemon working their magic.
5. Rinse your body with luke warm water and enjoy your soft silky skin.

Get Shiny Hair With Argan Oil. Thousands of years ago the tribes of Morocco discovered something miraculous about the Argan Tree. They realized that the oil, which is extracted from its fruit, had the most amazing healing properties. Argan oil is made from the crushed kernels of the argan tree, which can only be found in Morocco. The fatty acids and vitamin E penetrate your hair, skin and nails to boost hydration and repair your cells.

Nourish Skin with Rhassoul-This reddish-brown clay is found only in the Atlas mountains of Morocco and has been used by Moroccan women for centuries to care for their skin and hair. Rhassoul is loaded with minerals that will feed and nourish the skin such as silicon, iron, magnesium, potassium, sodium, lithium, and trace elements. Combine the rhassoul clay with water and use as a soap, skin conditioner, shampoo, and facial and body mask.

They care. Probably the number one most important secret and aspect of Moroccan beauty is that they care about how they look and feel. Moroccan's believe that beauty is as much of a spiritual aspect as it is physical. They don't believe in quick fixes or easy solutions which is why they dedicate a lifetime to bathing their body with the utmost care and respect. Both the men and women take pride in beauty and take great care to use only the finest of natural products and ingredients. Their beauty products are derived from only the best of rare plants, herbs, spices and other things found within the land of Morocco, such as pure argan oil.

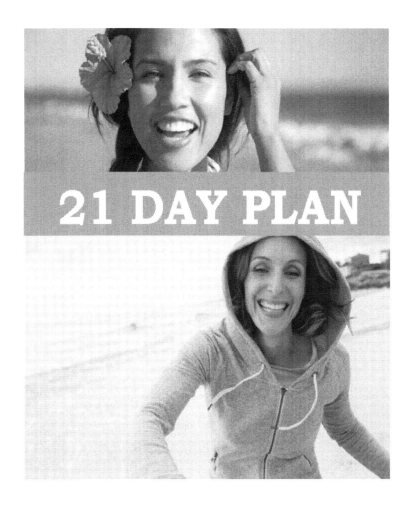

The idea behind a 21 day plan is to get you in the rhythm of looking after yourself. It takes three weeks to break habits and build a more positive plan. The must do's on this plan are:

1) Write down 3 things you're grateful for each day

2) Journal about 1 positive experience each day

3) Exercise every single day (it doesn't have to be hardcore)

4) 15 minutes of meditation daily (you don't have to be a seasoned yogi - just do your best)

5) Do one act of random kindness each day

So go buy yourself a diary and schedule in your activities. Use this book as a reference and try and schedule in as many of the treatments and tips in as you can. Here is a guide to help you out and give you a little inspiration for your first week.

Week One

MONDAY	6.30 Wake up with a cup of warm lemon water
	6.45 Do some exercise like walking, yoga or jogging
	7.30 Dry body brush for 5 minutes and have a shower
	8.00 Cleanse and moisturize face
	8.10 Give yourself a blow-dry and put on some simple makeup
	8.40am Make yourself a green juice or smoothie
	7.30pm Give yourself a scalp massage
	7.45pm Have a bath with Epsom salts and lavender

	8.15pm Rub coconut oil in hair to leave overnight for conditioning
TUESDAY	6.30am Wake up and do 15 minutes of meditation 7.00am Have a healthy breakfast of fresh seasonal fruit 7.30am Map your face and see what you can do to heal your skin disorders 7.40am Give yourself a face massage when doing your morning face routine 7.00pm Give yourself a manicure and paint your nails red or some other vibrant color 7.30pm Have a healing shower and cozy up in your favorite pajamas 8.00pm Sip on a herbal tea while you journal
WEDNESDAY	6.30am Go for an early morning walk and connect with nature and your surrounds 7.30am Make yourself a healthy smoothie – try the berry smoothie in this book

8.00am Give yourself a brow shape

8.30 Do a facial scrub

7.30pm Have a mud bath to purify

8.00pm Give yourself a pedicure

THURSDAY	6.30am Start the day off by reading something positive for 20 minutes 7.00am Do some light exercise to get your blood pumping and skin nourished 8.00am Give yourself a facial steam clean 7.30pm Make up a body scrub and polish your body to perfection 8.00pm Unwind with some mindful breathing whilst listening to some relaxing music
FRIDAY	6.30 am Greet the morning with a few yoga poses 7.00am Feed your body with a green juice or smoothie 7.30am Dare to wear some red lipstick and maybe some red shoes today. 8.00pm Focus on something that makes you unique. 7.30pm Spend the evening de-cluttering

a drawer, a room or your make-up bag

8.45pm Burn some lavender oil while you journal

SATURDAY	7.00am Go for a swim and feel the water gently rock your body
	8.00am Have a protein rich breakfast of either eggs on whole meal toast or a protein smoothie
	9.00am Do something that you have never done before.
	6.00pm Get ready for your night out by getting creative with a new make-up style – this is the night to re-invent yourself
	11.30pm make sure you wash your face before bed
SUNDAY	8.00am Start the morning with a few gentle stretches
	8.30am Have a relaxing bath and put on some comfortable clothes
	9.30 Have a nourishing vegetable juice.
	11.00 – 4.00pm Spend the day pampering yourself

This book is more than just a beauty book – it is a philosophy and a way of life. When you implement the tips and tools from this book into your own life you will empower yourself and feel amazing.

True beauty is the power to be you – remember it shines from the inside out. It is about confidence, kindness, passion, subtle enhancements and most of all accepting yourself for the way you are. The only way to connect with the divine beauty within yourself is to work it – just like a muscle it comes alive the more you pump it.

The one message I hope you take from this book is to totally appreciate, respect and honor yourself. Your life is constantly moving and evolving – your looks, your experiences, your wisdom and the people you meet. Remember that every stage of life is beautiful. Sometimes you just have to take a deep breath, relax and smile. After all a smile is a woman's best cosmetic.

Made in the USA
San Bernardino, CA
11 December 2013